RISE AND FALL OF MANAGED CARE: HISTORY OF THE MASS MEDICAL MOVEMENT

RISE AND FALL OF MANAGED CARE: HISTORY OF THE MASS MEDICAL MOVEMENT

RICHARD DEAN SMITH

Nova Science Publishers, Inc.
New York

Senior Editors: Susan Boriotti and Donna Dennis
Coordinating Editor: Tatiana Shohov
Office Manager: Annette Hellinger
Graphics: Wanda Serrano
Editorial Production: Jennifer Vogt, Matthew Kozlowski, Jonathan Rose and Maya Columbus
Circulation: Ave Maria Gonzalez, Vera Popovich, Luis Aviles, Melissa Diaz,
          Nicolas Miro and Jeannie Pappas
Communications and Acquisitions: Serge P. Shohov
Marketing: Cathy DeGregory

Library of Congress Cataloging-in-Publication Data

Smith, Richard Dean, 1931-
    The rise and fall of managed care: history of the mass medical movement / Richard Dean Smith.
    p. cm.
    Includes bibliographical references and index.
    ISBN 1-59033-306-3.
    1. Managed care plans (Medical care)—United States—History. 2. Health maintenance organizations—United States—History. I. Title.

RA413.5.U5 S654 2002
362.1'04258'0973—dc21

2002066019

Copyright © 2002 by Nova Science Publishers, Inc.
          400 Oser Ave, Suite 1600
          Hauppauge, New York 11788-3619
          Tele. 631-231-7269   Fax 631-231-8175
          e-mail: Novascience@earthlink.net
          Web Site: http://www.novapublishers.com

Printed in the United States of America

"You can diagnose a heresy," said the Frenchman, "by the passion with which it seeks converts. A subconscious knowledge of being hopelessly wrong compels you to find adherents who will assure you that you are right."

Erik Linklater. *The Dark of Summer* (1956)

CONTENTS

PREFACE

Decline in authority of religious institutions and power of the state during the humanistic movement gave rise to the modern invention of the individual, especially during eighteenth and nineteenth centuries. The individual, freed from constraints of church and community, found himself powerless as new poor from the country encountered the new rich in cities. Concurrent with appearance of the individual came the "age of the crowd" in collective behavior of individuals formed into masses following a leader or an idea.[1]

Individuals in a mass behave differently from individuals in isolation: sometimes in heroic, self-sacrificing actions, or in primitive, destructive behavior. When individuals form into a mass, the mass itself assumes its own character or personality.

Mass movements demonstrate certain general features depending on their underlying basic ideas: rational following reasonable principles, or irrational following an emotional and unreasonable path. Mass movements may work within existing norms of social boundaries and institutions, or discard all norms and institutions reversing direction in a complete reversal of values.

Characters play distinct roles in mass movements: zealots, men and women-of-letters, and practical men and women-of-action.

A rational, norm-oriented movement tends to be slowly progressive and advances according to reasonable demands for day-to-day change. An irrational,

---

[1] Serge Moscovici. *The Age of the Crowd: A Historical Treatise on Mass Psychology.* Translated by J.C. Whitehouse. Cambridge, London, New York, New Rochelle, Melbourne, and Sydney: Cambridge University Press, 1985. pp. 13-23.

concept-oriented mass movement tends to be sudden, emotional and driven by a vague promise of an idealized future.[2]

In considering changes in American medicine, claimed to be a 'revolution,' here we examine the nature of the mass movement into managed medical care, and compare it to behavior of other mass movements. Systematic study of mass movements dates only to 1895 in the works of Gustave Le Bon, a French physician, and by a number of additional social scientists during the 19th and 20th centuries. Similar mass movements occurred in academic and financial institutions concurrent with managed care.[3] By examining background, development, and implementation of mass movement into managed care, whether rational and norm-oriented or irrational and concept-oriented, and the characters involved, we may gain understanding about its history, its probable course and outcome.

---

[2] Eric Hoffer. *The True Believer: Thoughts on the Nature of Mass Movements*. New York: Harper & Row, 1951.

[3] Charles P. Kindleberger. *Manias, Panics, and Crashes: A History of Financial Crises*. New York and Chichester: John Wiley & Sons. 3rd Edition, 1996; Paul R. Gross and Norman Levitt. *Higher Superstition: The Academic Left and its Quarrels with Science*. Baltimore and London: The Johns Hopkins University Press, 1994.

Chapter I

THE BEGINNINGS

I. 1. INTRODUCTION

Since the early 1970s, rising medical costs resulted in a profusion of health care plans and criticism of the profession of medicine: a confusing, chaotic, divisive setting for providing medical care. Little or no communication took place between those who purchased medical insurance plans and those who provided medical services—physicians, dentists, hospitals, and other providers. Promotion of managed care plans took on an excited, carnival atmosphere generating promise that a glorious, new era was approaching.

Since doctors order most medical care, managed care proponents emphasized the importance of controlling practices of doctors. They claimed extensive changes were needed, that almost any criticism against the profession of medicine was warranted. Enterprising economists, entrepreneur consultants and a host of others became self-styled experts and advisers to hospitals and businesses over the issue of "cost containment" and invented the imperative "runaway costs." Accusations leveled against physicians by advocates of managed care were puzzling, disturbing, and frustrating. We were told that "managed care is what's out there," "business likes managed care," and managed care is "here to stay." The new ethic became marketplace competition, cost containment, prevention, and control.

Although most doctors at one time objected to the idea of managed care, rising sentiment against regular fee-for-service practice eventually took its toll to the point many physicians became convinced that it was up to doctors to make managed care work. Corporate benefits managers at first were opposed to the notion of managed care, but gave in to pressure from corporate management.

Managed care advocates created fear, uncertainty, and division by telling physicians that the only possibility of survival in "changing climate of health care" was to "embrace" managed care. Economists and politicians charging outright criminal activity by all physicians became the norm. Doctors and public were told that a new age had dawned, the old order was out, we had better get on board or be left behind. By declaring managed care an "unassailable truth," managed care was propelled into a revolution, a mass movement. Yet, physicians who "embraced" managed care found themselves in an ethical and practical bind.

Enthusiasm that led to the managed care mass movement followed the same course as other mass movements—a restructuring of medical care was called for, the old was suddenly outdated, a "crisis" proclaimed, a social transformation declared!

I. 2. BACKGROUND

Medical insurance, or health insurance, came into being during the Great Depression as a way to prevent hospital closures with establishment of the first hospital plan in 1936 and coverage for surgical fees in 1940 by Blue Cross and Blue Shield. In 1937, contractor Henry Kaiser started a pre-paid health plan to serve workers at Kaiser Industries. The Kaiser *Permanente* Health Plan formed in 1945 enrolling employees from non-Kaiser industries.

By 1952, health insurance entered into politics, but not until 1965 was major health care legislation passed in Title XVIII Medicare, and Title IXX Medicaid which provided health insurance for 20 percent of the population, and 25 percent by 2000. With expansion of health insurance during the 1950s and 1960s, both private and public, demand for medical services increased rapidly. Cost of medical care increased more rapidly than the cost of living.

Traditional reimbursement methods, fee-for-service for physicians and cost reimbursement for hospitals, were seen as culprits and became the focus of medical insurance "reform." Claims were made that financial incentives of physicians reinforced demands and expectations of anxious patients. Prestige of costly technology, liability-induced defensive medicine, and government-sponsored proliferation of health care personnel—especially physicians—added to criticism about rising medical costs.

During middle decades of the twentieth century, progress in medical care came with exciting frequency. New treatments, such as insulin, thyroid hormone, penicillin, and new anesthesia and surgery, were dramatic in their effects and ability to save and sustain life. Progress did not necessarily result in lower costs, but productivity by business employees was often related to the effectiveness of medical treatment. After World War II, interest in matters of health and medical care grew enormously. Biomedical research on major diseases was supported generously by private donations, venture capital, and public grants.

While Medicare kept its promise for decades, problems were apparent from the beginning with Medicaid (Medi-cal in California) which came about in 1967 with the slogan, "to get the poor into the mainstream of medicine"—that is, fee-for-service medical practice—and seen as a public benefit. Medicaid was to pay 80 percent of prevailing hospital and physician charges. Within six months, enrollment in Medicaid exceeded government estimates by 30 percent! Since patients on Medicaid are by definition in need of medical services large amounts of services were provided by fee-for-service physicians and hospitals at little or no compensation, or at a loss.

For three decades, "highest-quality care for all" dominated health care policy. Not surprisingly, spending for health care increased from under 5% of the Gross Domestic Product in 1950s to more than 11% by the late 1980s. In addition, after 1980, a large proportion of health care resources went to marketing, advertising, computer systems, and management consulting.[1] Health entitlements grew as the disabled, those on kidney dialysis, and others became beneficiaries of Medicare in 1972. The number of patients covered by Medicare and Medicaid grew faster than the population covered by private health insurance, especially after 1988. Hospitals over-charged regular insurance plans to pay for Medicaid shortfall, called 'pass through costs,' 'cost shifting,' or free-riding, which increased the cost of medical insurance. Subsequently, additional health plans began to reimburse hospitals below costs resulting in more cost shifting.

In the early 1970s, "cost crisis" was assumed to be due to "faulty incentives" embodied in "faulty institutional structures" that could be reorganized by a "market discipline" of prepayment, and that group practice would produce greater efficiency: that vigorous price competition would result in new system-wide "efficiencies and cost-containment." By a factory-like or production-line practice of medicine, managed care or "HMOs" were declared to be "self-regulating entities" through market forces eliminating "undesirable side effects" and would produce "improved quality, increased access, and lower costs" without the assumed incentives in fee-for-service, third-party-payment.[2]

The Department of Health, Education and Welfare (HEW) looked for a solution that would satisfy its critics in business on medical costs. To dismay of

---

[1] V.R. Fuchs. "The 'Competition Revolution' in Health Care." *Health Affairs* 7 Summer (1988) 5-24.
[2] Lawrence D. Brown. *Politics and Health Care Organization: HMOs as Federal Policy.* Washington, DC: The Brookings Institution, 1983, pp. 17-18.

the medical profession, President Nixon's administration endorsed the concept of prepaid group practice as its policy for slowing the rate of increase in health care expenditures. President Nixon's understanding of and involvement in the HMO deliberations was, as an observer recalled, "virtually nil."[3] A Republican administration worked with Democrat legislators to enact the Health Maintenance Organization Act of 1973.[4] In the process, they advocated Kaiser *Permanente* in California: Kaiser *Permanente* was declared to provide "high quality service at a low cost." What followed became a complex, bizarre assortment of competing managed care plans.

Private fee-for-service practice of medicine came under attack: doctors were held to the standard of managed care in Kaiser *Permanente*. Doctors' efforts to be heard were ignored as self-serving in the clamor for managed care, since doctors, by a strange logic, were declared "cost unconscious." Once endorsed, managed care plans grew from 30 plans in 1970 to over 600 by 1995. For-profit managed care HMOs were presented to public and profession as being successful, rich and powerful.

Although advances in anesthesia and surgical techniques occurred in the eighteenth and nineteenth centuries, and many disease processes were beginning to be understood, none of the advances had any real effect on life expectancy. However, to effectiveness of social and economic circumstances on health and longevity of people, we must now add new life-saving drugs and medical treatments, which entail increased costs.

Fee-for-service practice disappeared as patients were moved into managed care plans by employers and by government. Subsequently, daily medical practice decisions were made by employees of managed care companies resulting in growing hostility from the public, and divisiveness among doctors. Morale suffered, doctors grew angry, defensive, fearful, and eventually—silent.

Cynicism reigned: medicine was conceived as a simple, mechanistic undertaking that could be put into an assembly line—a simplistic notion, based on primary care, anti-specialist, and anti-intellectual ideas. The "preferred provider" concept arose 1982 in that Blue Cross was able to reduce the number of doctors on its list by designating physicians who were willing to accept significantly lower payments in order to be regarded as "preferred" in order to retain patients.

While Medicare is often cited as a serious problem, Medicare became one of the most successful public programs: Medicare succeeded beyond anyone's expectations. The control of many acute and fatal illnesses produced a growing

[3] Brown. p. 219.
[4] John K. Iglehart. "Health Policy Report: The American Health Care System." *New England Journal of Medicine* 327 (1992) 742-747.

elderly and advanced elderly population for the first time in human history. The elderly suffer more chronic disorders, which require care, but cannot be cured or eliminated. In addition, large numbers of the elderly experience tragic degenerative diseases of multiple organ systems.

Not all of the rise in life expectancy can be attributed to improved and more effective medical care. Medical services depend on a sound economy and a secure political environment—the problem of cost of health care occurs only in stable, affluent countries. Add to that current public health and preventive measures, effective treatments of illnesses that carried away the elderly in former centuries, the current generation may expect to become ninety-year olds, or older.

"Reforms" of medicine by managed care were based almost entirely on care of acute illnesses, but in the matter of chronic disorders, managed care emphasized limiting access to medical services. If a health plan became proficient at treating a chronic disorder, plan managers were concerned that public knowledge of its expertise would result in "adverse selection" resulting in higher utilization of health care resources. Managed care plans were based on the control of financial resources; health plan managers discouraged dissemination of effective treatment information that might attract high-cost populations. Managed care plans labeled such information proprietary so that it would not lead to higher utilization which would be financially disastrous.[5]

A new ethic developed on strength of relentless pressuring of business and government to "embrace" managed care with claims of a new set of powerful influences, such as price competition, drive for market share, assumption of insurance risk by providers, impact of investment capital, and new roles of employers and patients. Additional financial burden accrued by an enormous rise in administrative costs within managed care companies, hospitals, and doctors' offices. Administrative costs do not provide services or produce revenue, but are costs that cannot be recovered elsewhere, such as increased legal costs complying with regulations, dealing with managed care companies, medical staff legal costs, and hospital legal costs. The financial stakes were enormous.[6]

From point of view of the managed care industry, doctors, hospitals, and other providers had an "incentive" to maximize the extent, sophistication, and intensity of treatment, or "cost-plus" medical care which was thought to cause cost escalation, and was criticized as causing "supplier-induced demand," where

---

[5] Robert G. Frank. "Lessons from the Great Battle: Health Care Reform, 1992-1994." *Archives of Physical Medicine and Rehabilitation.* 78 (1997) 120-124.

[6] Lynn Etheredge, Stanley B. Jones, and Lawrence Lewin. "What Is Driving Health System Change?" *Health Affairs* 15 (1996) winter 93-104.

the sellers of services helped to create demand for services they provided.[7] To illustrate the conflict further, Congressman George Miller of California avowed that medical care became "the fourth necessity."

A mass movement, such as managed care, infects people with a malady and creates a demand for change.[8]

I. 3. DEFINITION OF MANAGED MEDICAL CARE

Managed care was characterized as a system that integrated financing and delivery of medical care: contracts with selected physicians and hospitals that provided medical care services to enrolled members for a set monthly premium; utilization and quality controls that contracting providers agreed to accept; financial incentives for patients to use providers and facilities associated with the plan; and assumption of financial risk by doctors. Thus, physicians' role was altered from agent for patients' welfare to a conflicting need for cost control—from advocacy to allocation.[9] Managed care's central tenet was that doctors, hospitals, and patients couldn't be trusted to prescribe medical treatment: outside supervision was needed—not only to hold down costs, but also to decide what constituted appropriate care. Old incentives that supposedly encouraged excessive, unnecessary care would be replaced by rewarding thrift, and punishing "overtreatment."[10]

Capitation payment, or set fee, was paid per person per month for whatever medical care they received during a defined period of time, usually one year, but sometimes six months when contracts were renewed and adjusted like other insurance plans. Capitation had a number of synonyms, such as "health maintenance organization" or "HMO," integrated systems, and numerous other variations that deal with managed care companies. Some were traditional insurance companies; others were money handling entities involved with health care. The public was tempted by the notion that managed care companies offered 'something for nothing' in that the patient paid a set fee and if costs went over that amount, doctors and hospitals paid the rest.

[7] Victor Tabbuch and Gerald Swanson. "Changing Paradigms in Medical Payment." *Archives of Internal Medicine* 156 (1996) 357-360.
[8] Eric Hoffer. *The True Believer: Thoughts on the Nature of Mass Movements.* New York: Harper & Row, 1952, p. 55.
[9] Iglehart.
[10] George Anders. *Health Against Wealth: HMOs and the Breakdown of Medical Trust.* Boston and New York: Houghton Mifflin, 1996, pp. 25-26.

Proponents of managed care claimed that incentives encouraged providers to operate efficiently within the amount of time and money available in addition to providing high-quality care. Patients received a health plan, which covered specified health care services, regardless of number of visits or procedures performed. Proponents asserted that physicians also had an incentive to provide preventive services to decrease incidence and severity of illnesses, which would result in better care to consumers on the assumption that prevention lowers costs.

Americans were expected to abruptly adjust to a system that inverted traditional medical care ethics and recast doctors as double agents.[11] Ideally, integration of hospitals, physicians, and all other providers would join to accomplish a shared goal, learn to create efficient governance, to align incentives, and to manage risks so the system could care for a population at a predetermined price while making necessary services available to all and preserving or improving quality of care.[12]

Others said that managed care was the "blunt instrument" payers chose to change the culture of medicine. The issue of appropriateness—an underlying factor in use of technology and its inherently higher costs—was accompanied by attention to cost-effectiveness. The overriding issue of the managed care industry was its claim of effectiveness in controlling costs.

A pool of money was set aside by managed care companies for hospital inpatient services or referrals to specialists. If money remained in the pool at the end of the year, it was to be shared by the managed care company and its physicians, such as Kaiser *Permanente's* "unspent surplus" which at one time amounted to approximately 30 to 50 percent of physicians' base salary. The surplus created an incentive not to refer patients for care, with the risk that primary care doctors handled complex cases and difficult problems that used to be referred to specialists.[13] Managed care advocates declared the advantages of "preventive care, not unnecessary care." The slogan "runaway costs" became the emotional catalyst behind sanction of managed care without regard to causes of rising costs.

Managed care was promoted on cynicism toward patients and criticism of physicians.

---

[11] Iglehart.

[12] A.S. Relman. "Controlling Costs by 'Managed Competition'—Would It Work? *New England Journal of Medicine* 328 (1993) 133-135.

[13] "Background Paper for Capitation Hearing." California Legislature. Senate Committee on Judiciary. Senator Charles M. Calderon, Chairman.

I. 4. CRITICISM OF PHYSICIANS

The managed care mass movement derived its force from the criticism of practicing fee-for-service physicians, such that the profession of medicine experienced criticism from all sides. That the physician-patient relationship had deteriorated became part of dogma of "reform." If literature is a guide, the physician-patient relationship has not deteriorated because it was always in doubt; a few samples illustrate:

In Anthony Trollope's novel *Doctor Thorne* (1858), the competition between Doctor Thorne and his rival, satirically called Doctor Fillgrave, is the focus of the story. With a slovenly manner, Doctor Thorne is a poor man: "the gift of saving money had not been his." The wealthy families of Barsetshire capriciously dismiss one doctor to call in the other.

Robert Burn's poem "Death and Doctor Hornbook" (1787), illustrates:

'That's just a swatch o' Hornbook's way,
'Thus goes he on from day to day,
'Thus does he poison, kill, an' slay,
            'An's weel paid for't;
'Yet stops me o' my lawfu' prey,
            'Wi his damn'd dirt!

Chaucer's fourteenth-century Doctour of Physik in *The Canterbury Tales* is suspected of being something of a humbug, in league with his apothecaries to fleece the public.[14] Even though medicine today is far removed from practice of the days of Chaucer, character traits of his physician are amazingly similar to current criticism against doctors. A few centuries later, Shakespeare's physicians were satirized and comical. Boccaccio (1313-1375) was equally critical of doctors, as well as lawyers, clerics, and academics.

During the Islamic Renaissance of the ninth century, physician al-Ruhawi wrote in *Adab al-Tabib,* or *Practical Medical Ethics:* "How many people hate physicians and execrate them instead of loving and respecting them since they hold them back from their desires and warn them not to follow their pleasures."[15]

When today's critics defame doctors, or when tenured economists derided the profession, they repeat what has been said about the profession for millennia using the theme of criticism to justify their own purposes.

---

[14] W.C. Curry. *Chaucer and the Mediaeval Sciences.* New York: Barnes and Noble, 1960.
[15] R.D. Smith. "*Adab al-Tabib*: Practical Medical Ethics of the Ninth Century." *ACCMA Bulletin.* Feb. 1982, p. 21.

In the mid-twentieth century, medicine received uncharacteristic sanction and support which is atypical in the history of medicine. A career in medicine offered promise of economic certainty or at least making a living; such is not the case through much of history. Those who are healthiest complain the most, but those who are ill and have greatest contact with physicians and have substantial medical bills complain least and are the most appreciative.

Nevertheless, some journalists allowed no exceptions by generalizing from the particular to the general, claiming that "unscrupulous doctors" increased their incomes by any excuse in the "sins of fee-for-service medicine...to jack up revenue,"[16] an *argumentum ad odium*, from enmity, malice. Some claimed that "unsupervised" fee-for-service medicine was "deeply flawed" giving rise to the managed care mass movement. To critics, over-treatment was inevitable if doctors and hospitals were paid a fee for each exam, test, or surgery.[17] Such complaints against physicians are not new, but follow the historical tradition of physician criticism. Parallels of managed care with nineteenth-century quackery are striking: orthodox physicians felt besieged by the growing nostrum business, burgeoning competing systems, and declining public confidence. Nostrum vendors denounced restrictions on their unorthodoxy as a "wicked monopoly" for the benefit of doctors.[18]

Complaints against physicians show little change over the ages. Mass movements do not require the existence of a deity, ideal or truth, but it must believe in a 'devil', which gives the movement its greatest strength: the devil must be vivid and tangible. In the case of the managed care mass movement, it was doctors in general and, more specifically, those in fee-for-service practice of medicine who were the mass movement's 'necessary devil.' Hatred, enmity, is the most accessible and comprehensive unifying agent to a cause generating a feeling of kinship. Self-contempt of adherents transforms into a hatred of others. It is easier to hate an enemy with much good to its credit, such as regular fee-for-service practicing physicians, than one that is all bad. The mass movement seeks, and deserves, the hatred of its 'devil,' which tends to give sanction and lends support to the claims of superiority of the mass movement. Enmity gives meaning and purpose to an empty life; a mass movement nurtures a fanatical grievance. The undercurrent of admiration in hatred manifests itself in the inclination to

---

[16] Anders. p. 247.
[17] Anders. p. 251.
[18] James Harvey Young. *American Health Quackery*. Princeton, New Jersey: Princeton University Press, 1992, p. 44.

imitate those who are hated; every mass movement shapes itself after its specific 'devil.'[19]

Fee-for-service medical practice, or other systems of medical practice, offered no holy cause to cling to and no corporate whole for masses to be engulfed in. Criticizing and demonizing doctors and denunciation of regular practice of medicine became a necessary ingredient in the mass movement into managed care.

---

[19] Hoffer. pp. 87,90.

Chapter II

EXPANSION

II. 1. GROWTH OF MANAGED MEDICAL CARE

The Knox-Keene Act (1975) required all companies with over twenty-five employees to offer a managed care plan whether or not companies agreed with doctrines of managed care. The appearance of one managed care company stimulated rise of others. Mergers of managed care companies gave the impression that larger managed care companies became ever more powerful. Managed care companies increased non-medical services burden, but this increase in costs did not influence its growth and expansion. Arguments for and against managed care became irrelevant as managed care gained momentum to the exclusion of regular fee-for-service medical practice or other forms of medical financing.

To business, benefits managers, and the bottom line, the claims presented by the managed care industry were appealing, especially to boards of directors of corporations and to stockholders. In the mid-1980s, faced with intensified global competition and "uncontrollable health care costs," employer-purchasers of health care encouraged their employees to join managed care plans. Long term effects of their decisions in health care do not enter into corporate planning. The shift of employees into managed care gained little notice; exaggerated claims convinced profit-oriented executives. Business was satisfied that managed care had emerged as the "dominant model" of American health care system on vague promises of future rewards. Business groups assumed that managed care plans were the only option and looked no further: short-term cost and only cost dominated their decisions. Apprehensions of business about the effect of health care costs on success of their businesses came to the fore.

Momentum toward managed care gained even as criticism arose. Patients and doctors were swept up in managed care plans that were poorly defined and poorly understood, but highly promoted. An urgency, a disquiet that much was amiss provoked mistrust and uneasiness in the minds of the public, business, and government, yet convinced of a vague, exaggerated promise of future savings. By 1997, managed care plans provided coverage for 77 percent of Americans and their dependents who were insured through their employers. In addition, 80,000 elderly Americans switched to Medicare managed care each month largely because of an appearance of cost savings.

Managed care strategy claimed to control health care costs in the United States by assuming the need to do something about increased medical costs but with the desire to avoid governmental or central administration. Federal policymakers seized on a "seemingly painless, inexpensive, nondepriving, nonconflictual, and nonregulatory approach." Managed care would challenge fee-for-service practice in marketplace competition. Claims by advocates of managed care on supposed virtues of HMOs—efficiency, competition, and choice—proved irresistible to policy makers of the early 1970s, and "they embraced the HMO strategy warmly."[1]

The mass movement into managed care was well under way. All forms of dedication, devotion, loyalty and self-surrender become a clinging to something which might give worth and meaning to ease frustration. "Embracing" a substitute necessarily must be passionate and extreme—faith in the mass movement must be extravagant and uncompromising. Mass movements regard antagonists as potential converts to their own cause. Mass movements are competitive, in that a gain in adherents by one mass movement results in a loss to another mass movement, and that mass movements are interchangeable, such as managed care advocates and consultants with their checkered employment histories who move from one cause to another.[2]

Every mass movement has its distant hope, an intoxicant or opiate to suppress impatience and to reconcile the masses to their lot. A mass movement attracts and holds adherents not by its doctrine or promises, but by refuge it offers from anxieties, barrenness and meaninglessness of individual existence. Misfits find meaning in a separation from self, and by losing themselves in the close collectivity of a mass movement.[3]

[1] Lawrence D. Brown. *Politics and Health Care Organization: HMOs as Federal Policy.* Washington, DC: The Brookings Institution, 1983, pp. 492-493.
[2] Eric Hoffer. *The True Believer: Thought on the Nature of Mass Movements.* New York: Harper & Row, 1951. pp. 25-26.
[3] Hoffer. pp. 35, 44, 50.

II. 2. ENTHUSIASM

Excitement generated by advocates of the managed care industry overcame objections and opposition: a new era was proclaimed! Patients, businesses, insurance companies, doctors, hospitals, and investors were caught in enthusiasm for the managed care mass movement as the new wave, a new solution, a new way to practice medicine—a *revolution*! Journals and magazines that advise doctors on financial and practice matters said the movement could not be resisted, to do so meant certain failure, and that the best way to deal with the future of medical practice was to go "wholly into managed care." The more a doctor might consider alternatives increased the likelihood of being left out while other doctors would get managed care contracts and survive in an "increasingly competitive health care arena." So far reaching and so insistent were harangues to physicians, to patients, and to business that only a few are given here, but illustrate the pressure and enthusiasm.

In 1992, advocates claimed that managed care was clearly a phenomenon that was "here to stay" despite reluctance of doctors. In addition, most legislative proposals on health care promoted expansion of managed care.[4] An era dominated by independent solo medical practitioners was said to be ending. Within another decade, managed care advocates claimed that practicing physicians would belong to organized groups of providers to deliver medical services on a capitated basis.

Business reporters for newspaper advocated a "production-line" model of medical practice: "factory-like efficiency" to routine aspects of medicine with claims that managed care would reduce health care costs up to 20% and slow further increases. Or that managed care's triumph over fee-for-service practice was "stunning." Managed care was presented to the public as a chance of a lifetime, an unusual opportunity that may not come again. Limited enrollment periods gave a sense of urgency making decisions to join managed care plans less likely to be carefully considered. For some, managed care was a gamble, a chance to defy the odds, and they "embraced" managed care readily.

Rapid shifts occurred in the health care system, such as growth of managed care organizations and for-profit hospital chains which became even larger through mergers and acquisitions. Not-for-profit hospitals and insurance companies converted to for-profit status. The number of physicians in solo practice diminished, and Medicare beneficiaries signed up in large numbers with managed care plans. Academic medical centers scrambled to develop integrated,

---

[4] John K. Iglehart. "Health Policy Report: The American Health Care System." *New England Journal of Medicine* 327 (1992) 742-747.

managed care systems and to organized their physicians into physician-hospital organizations: a mass movement!

In the formation of mass movements, psychological processes run counter to the development of individual personality: in the mass, single individuals present themselves as uniform whether patients, physicians, or businesses. They were impelled to seek uniformity by urgings that had previously been denied from satisfaction, and multitudes of like-minded people gave support. Mass movements have many typical characteristics: the gradual continuous process of individual maturation is disrupted by identifying with and incorporating ideas of the mass. Conflicts between old and new are resolved by discarding old identifications and patterns of thought in favor of new mass slogans. Abrupt change of identification places the person under a control alien to himself and leads to decline in discriminating intelligence. Individual characteristics are swept aside in favor of mass aims; the individual is deflected from his own aim—that of developing an independent self, which only a short time before had seemed to the individual and to society the highest ideal of human maturity.[5]

Adherents to a mass movement must have blind faith in omnipotence of its doctrine.[6] Proselytizing is more an impassioned search for something not yet found than for something already present, a search for a demonstration of an absolute truth and the only truth, attested by such statements that "managed care is here to stay." Those movements with the greatest conflict between profession and practice, associated with strong feelings of guilt, are likely to be the most ardent in imposing the movement on others.[7]

The zealot is convinced that the cause of the mass movement is massive, permanent and eternal—a "rock of ages." A sense of security is derived from passionate attachment, not from claims of excellence of the cause. The zealot is not a stickler for principle: he embraces a cause not because of its justness and worthiness but because of his desperate need for something to hold on to.[8] A mass movement's call for action evokes an eager response in the frustrated, for they see in action a cure for all that ails them with self-forgetting and gives a sense of purpose and worth.[9]

By developing a program of publicity, demonizing doctors, and stimulating open conflict in order to dramatically, and substantially alter the movement's

[5] Max Hernandez. "Group Formation and Ideology. Text and Context." *International Journal of Psycho-Analysis* 69 (1988) 163-170.
[6] Hoffer. p. 17.
[7] Hoffer. pp. 102-103.
[8] Hoffer. pp. 80-81.
[9] Hoffer. p. 112.

relation to its society, the mass movement of managed care endeavored to capture the society with a full-time corps of members dedicated to managed care. The investment of much of the movement's resources went to expand the number of dedicated members, and to generate large-scale funds. The image of a well funded, undivided dedication to furthering the movement's position towards managed care enabled the dedicated to carry on by an expanding body of true believers.[10]

The Nixon administration's managed care proposal was described as a "textbook example of how an executive initiative ought *not* to be constructed." HMOs entered the legislative agenda abruptly in 1970 when the concept was "embraced" by Department of Health, Education and Welfare (HEW) generalists without background in health policy issues who knew little about managed care or HMOs, but were attracted by what HMOs would *not* entail. They relied on a highly abstract model of HMO "proincentive" and "self-regulating" assumptions while ignoring questions and reservation of HEW specialists and Prepaid Group Practice representatives. Soon after the HMO initiative had been adopted, those at HEW, led by Secretary Richardson who was equally lacking in knowledge the workings of prepaid group practice, convinced the White House that an aggressive effort to develop HMOs would "save money, reinvigorate competition in the health care system, avoid regulation, and meet the needs of underserved areas." All of these claims were "conjectural and unsubstantiated; some were far fetched indeed."

After the president had enthusiastically endorsed HMOs and an administration bill sent to Congress, those at HEW finally gave the proposal some detailed thought. The Nixon HMO proposal grew out of "HEW entrepreneurship, with little discussion and less clarity." After commitment had been made to managed care and legislation introduced, "institutional involvement grew and deliberation proceeded."[11] Strained and deteriorating relations between legislative and executive branches were constant during 1970-1973. Although some important legislation emerged, "None, however, was surrounded by the aura of pervasive misunderstanding and failure that assailed the HMO law."[12] The HMO law was alien to the department's general experience, and resulted largely from a distrust of the HEW's administrative capacity and responsibility.[13]

---

[10] John Lofland. Chapter 14 "White-Hot Mobilization: Strategies of a Millenarian Movement." in James L. Wood and Maurice Jackson. *Social Movements: Development, Participation, and Dynamics*. Belmont, CA: Wadsworth, 1982, pp. 221-228.
[11] Brown. pp. 269-270.
[12] Brown. p. 272.
[13] Brown. pp. 280-281.

Following the subconscious instincts of mass behavior, the mass movement or revolution into the managed care was based on illusion and error.

II. 3. PROMISE OF AN EXCEPTIONAL RETURN—GREED

Managed care was urged on doctors as a way to survive the "revolution." Health care consultants appealed to the motive of greed, that Medicare managed care offered doctors a chance to make "lots, *lots* of money." The medical profession faced an ethical and economic conflict of "unprecedented proportions" in a health care system that became a vast and highly lucrative marketplace.

Managed care companies served motives of greed and avarice of CEOs, executives, sales personnel of the managed care industry who regarded patients as "revenue producing biological preparations." In 1994, Health System International reportedly had $475 million in cash and grew at $500,000 a day; that the nine biggest HMOs had $9.5 billion in cash, i.e. bank deposits and marketable securities. Kaiser *Permanente* claimed reserves of $1.7 billion, and that US Healthcare had $1.16 billion in reserves. In 1994, publicly traded HMOs completed 13 acquisitions totaling almost $4 billion.

The effect on Wall Street was equally forceful: investment capital destabilized the status quo to gain excess profits throughout the health care system. Investment capital was attracted to relentless growth in managed care revenues and profits, thus creating a voracious appetite for profits from mergers and acquisitions. In 1980, the chairman of INA Corporation candidly said that his company's interest in HMO activity was very simple: profit—and that managed care produced their highest rate of return, saying that as long as health care generated above average return on investment, they were going to invest in it.[14] Executive pay to officers of managed care companies "exploded" since 1990, much of it in long-term incentive awards. Many would pay off only if the HMO's stock prices rise to specified high levels. Managed care companies were big-time businesses, not quasi-charitable organizations.

Before long, voluntary hospitals began to behave like investor-owned hospitals. Philanthropy and community contributions, a mainstay of support when hospital costs were relatively low, were no longer of much financial assistance. Altruistic motives that formerly guided the decisions of voluntary hospital management gave way to primary concern for the bottom line. So great was avarice in the momentum of the managed care industry, that the public had only

---

[14] *New York Times* August 25, 1980.

the vaguest idea of what was being perpetrated in the name of profit. Salespeople had taken over health care: the name of the game was "greed."[15]

The new ethic and morality presented to doctors and hospitals became: how could the doctor keep this patient healthy longer to make more income because the doctor was capitated? How much care could be withheld? What could be gotten-away-with?

II. 4. THE HEALTH CARE CONSULTING INDUSTRY

The claim of a "health care crisis" gave rise to a new opportunity: the health care consulting industry. Glib, slick, masters of management-speak, health care consultants and economists became spokespersons for managed care, nearly always with transient employment histories. Health care consultants flocked to an opportunity created by confusion and fearfulness of public and profession, emphatically stating a disclaimer at beginning and again at end of their presentations.

Hospitals and provider groups hired strategy consultants, sometimes at fees of over $1 million. The usual advice was to become a more "integrated delivery system" either through acquisitions, mergers or joint ventures. Consultants recommended currently popular concepts such as economies of scale, merging, changing doctors' practice patterns, and rewarding frugal care with slogans like "build a critical mass" in negotiating with insurers and managed care plans. In many cases, mergers did not help hospitals lower costs, but resulted in bureaucratic gridlock. Some mergers were mistakes. When partners in mergers searched for ways to separate, the same consultants earned even more on "post-merger integration" in all industries.

Members of the health care consulting industry declared that all of the history of medicine was passé; that incentives were reversed 180 degrees—that established institutions and norms had to be destroyed. Hospital administrators should "rejoice at empty beds and quiet wards," and that "capitated lives" were the key to success, not care of patients.

The "key dynamic" was large providers assuming capitated risk for entire patient populations, utilizing the principle of "economy of scale" and that capitated financing was an "unassailable good." The inevitable result was that providers became afraid of "revenue lock-out," as large health systems "put the squeeze" on independent providers—an appeal to fearmongering, and playing to

---

[15] Samuel A. Brody. letter *New England Journal of Medicine* 336 (1997) 72.

the gallery. Traditional measures of success—high occupancy rates, more procedures—were "suddenly invalid." A mass movement deliberately depicts the present as mean and miserable compared to a vague promising future, a threshold to the millennium, it must turn its back on the past.[16]

Accomplishing the mission of "embracing" managed care was called a "Herculean Task," emphasizing the "enormity" of the task, that is, "you can't do it without us, and we are not cheap." By the error of *Self-Assumed Authority*, they advocated vertical integration "in the same blood line, if not the immediate family, of Kaiser *Permanente*." In their view, "Only the foundation, staff and equity models can successfully compete with the likes of Kaiser [*Permanente*] in the future; full ownership of physician practices." By a mass of empty slogans and clichés, *fallacy of imposter terms*, hasty generalization, irrelevant conclusion, speculation, and appeal to fancy, they claimed to know the future. They claimed that physicians were ready to "make the leap" from independence to full integration overnight, by the appeal to crowd psychology, the bandwagon effect of herd-behavior. Supposedly, the highest calling for health systems was to serve physicians by creating a safe harbor from the "coming storm," an appeal to fear. The challenge was to convince physicians to cast his or her lot with the health system by joining the mass movement.[17]

The total amount of health care consulting fees was unknown, but some have said privately that advising a mid-sized hospital could claim $500,000, or a large hospital over $1 million in fees. Advisory and consultant fees of $1 million were common. Nor was Kaiser *Permanente* able to control its health care consulting costs whose fees to the health care consulting industry reportedly resulted in billings of as much as $3 million per month.[18]

Economists gained an extraordinary presence in the debate on providing medical care services in the US. During the past 30 years, economists published thousands of empirical articles on various aspects of health and medical care.[19] Scholars concluded that not only do economists disagree sharply about policy-making, it is disgracefully easy for managed care companies to shop around for an economist to support their views—economists also disagree widely about basic economic facts. Economists' views on policy questions correspond more closely

---

[16] Hoffer. pp. 66-67.

[17] *To the Greater Good: Recovering the American Physician Enterprise. Governance Committee.* Advisory Board Company, 1995.

[18] Chris Rauber. "Kaiser executive who cut hospitals hangs up scalpel." *San Francisco Business Times.* June 6-12, 1997.

[19] Victor R. Fuchs. "Economics, Values, and Health Care Reform." *The American Economic Review* 86 (1996) 1-24. Reprint.

to their personal values than to factual assumptions. In other words, "mere facts don't change their mind on issues."[20]

In an often cited study on health care, economist Kenneth Arrow's "Uncertainty and the Welfare Economics of Medical Care" in *The American Economic Review* (1963) claims that special economic problems of medical care are due to the existence of uncertainty in incidence of disease and in effectiveness of treatment. A transfer of purchasing power from the well to the ill increases demand for medical services which manifests itself in the short run by an increase in price of medical services and in the long run in an increase in the amount supplied. Arrow holds that virtually all the special features of provision of medical services stems from the prevalence of uncertainty, and that the most distinguishing characteristics of an individual's demand for medical services is that demand is not steady, but irregular and unpredictable. Except for preventive services, medical services result in satisfaction only in event of illness which is a departure from the normal state of health. In the case of medical care, product and activity of production are identical. The customer or patient cannot test the product or service before consuming it.

Arrow emphasized the importance of trust in the relation between patient and physician: the ethical restrictions on physicians are severe, and physicians' behavior is governed by a concern for "customer's" welfare, which would not be expected of a salesman. A 'collectivity-orientation' distinguishes medicine and other professions from business where self-interest on part of business participants is accepted norm; advice given by physicians as to further treatment by himself or others divorced from self-interest is dictated by objective needs of the case and not by financial considerations. Arrow says that ethical compulsion is not as absolute in practice as it is in theory which influences allocation of health care resources, as illustrated by the existence of charity treatment because of a tradition of human right to adequate medical care. Communicable diseases provide an obvious example of non-market interactions.[21] In medicine, demand will always exceed supply and administrative costs and the profit motive of managed care companies appeared uncontrollable.

A basic principle of economics is the "law of diminishing marginal returns" in the production model of industry. Claims of the relation of health out-comes to more in-hospital days for a patient with a given diagnosis, or number of diagnostic tests, or health status was challenged by economists and other managed

---

[20] Jonathan Marshall. "Economists Can't Seem to Agree on Anything." *San Francisco Chronicle* August 25, 1997.

[21] Kenneth J. Arrow. "Uncertainty and the Welfare Economics of Medical Care." *The American Economic Review* 53 (1963) 941-973.

care advocates: "…a great deal of 'flat-of-the-curve medicine' is being practiced in the United States today—that is, applications of health-care resources yielding no discernible or valuable health benefit."[22] In the "production model" of industry, an increase in spending should increase production and profit, an "up-slope of the curve." When an increase in spending is not followed by an increase in result or profit, the economists call the "flat of the curve." Analytical methods used to increase efficiency in industrial production when applied to medical care have not met with approval except by some economists and managed care enthusiasts who claim that medicine is no different than automobile assembly, grain growing, or computer-chip fabrication no matter what doctors and patients may think.[23]

In the case of acute illnesses, resources allocated are comparable to the up-slope of the curve in that an increase in expenditures results in better outcomes or production. The "flat of the curve" occurs in the case chronic diseases in which more money is spent without a greater ability of the individual to produce in the usual sense, such as diabetes, congestive heart failure, and other chronic diseases. A more problematic situation occurs in the case of terminal care or palliative care in which a *decrease* in the ability of the patient to produce occurs even though a great deal more resources are expended in medical care, which is comparable to a "decline of the curve." In this case, resources committed to care do not maintain the status quo, but slow the decline of the chronically ill consuming large amounts of medical care by those who often can not contribute to the general welfare or maintain even a minimal standard of self-care. "Decline of the curve" does not occur in an industrial production-model because once a machine costs more to operate than it produces in profit and can't be fixed, it is discarded.

The principal activity of the health care consulting industry was to beguile the gullible, benefiting no one except the peddler-consultants. Nevertheless, physicians and hospitals desperately reached out to the health care consulting industry to resolve their dilemmas, relying on doubtful authorities.

In sum, the consulting industry displayed the *Self-Trumpeter's Fallacy* of over-rated pretensions to superior intelligence whose assertions are to be deemed equivalent to truth–with a disclaimer. The absurdity that marks the general beliefs embraced by mass movements has never been an obstruction to their triumph; in

[22] A.C. Enthoven. "Shattuck Lecture—Cutting Cost Without Cutting Quality of Care." *New England Journal of Medicine* 298 (1978) 1229-1238.
[23] George Anders. *Health Against Wealth: HMOs and the Breakdown of Medical Trust.* Boston and New York: Houghton Mifflin, 1996, p. 40.

fact, the rhetoric and slogans of a mass movement must offer "some mysterious absurdity."[24]

II. 5. THE PRESS

Almost every publication that comments on medical care carried articles promoting managed care. During HMO open enrollment periods, daily newspapers published special sections with titles, such as "Which HMO is Right For You?" On September 22, 1997, the *San Francisco Chronicle* ran a six-page special section devoted to managed care with the headline "Which managed medical care plan for you?" These extra sections of free promotion and advertising for the managed care industry offered no balanced reporting by a similar six page supplement on the advantages of traditional fee-for-service, indemnity health insurance plans, or any other sort of plan. Exaggerated reports and slanted reporting provided the managed care industry with extensive, expensive free advertising and press sanction.

For forty years, Kaiser *Permanente* did not advertise except in its very early days. In the 1990s, Kaiser *Permanente* resorted to newspaper, radio, and television advertising; previously advertising was not necessary since newspapers and magazines reported alleged advantages of managed care in the form of Kaiser *Permanente* at no cost to Kaiser *Permanente* and it had no competition. Complaints to the press by physicians met with indifference or arrogance.

In 1970, the *Scientific American* published "The Delivery of Medical Care" by a Kaiser *Permanente* official which undermines existing norms with exaggerated claims and errors, such as emotive words, *Imputation of Bad Design*, *argumentum ad judicum* or Sham distinctions, vague generalities, *Self-Assumed Authority*, *argumentum ad metus* or fear, *argumentum ad imaginationem*, an appeal to fancy, the *Self-Trumpeter's Fallacy*, etc. Patients were to be sorted by an assembly line, production model by non-physician personnel using machines and technological devices that was claimed to save on costs.

In 1980, the editors of *Scientific American* were on the bandwagon with an article titled, "Health Maintenance Organizations" saying that Kaiser *Permanente* and Group Health Cooperative of Puget Sound "inspired" the Nixon

---

[24] Gustave Le Bon. *The Crowd: A Study of the Popular Mind.* (1895) Dunwoody, GA: Norman S. Berg, 2nd ed. 1984, p. 147.

administration to endorse "Health Maintenance Organization," which they call a "promotional term," based on:

1. Defined population and membership [selection].
2. Payment in advance made periodically [capitation].
3. Services provided by HMO physicians with outside specialists controlled by the HMO [rationing].
4. Voluntary enrollment by each individual or family [coercion by company benefits managers].

It lauds the alleged "cost-saving potential of competition," a failed concept. By the errors of *Self-Trumpeter's fallacy* and *paradoxical assertion*, the absurd is made to sound rational.

And in 1992, *Scientific American*'s "Health Care Reform" used *emotive words*: "severely flawed," "the costs of health care have exploded," "escalating costs," etc. to make its claim for managed care and health care "reform." Then contradicts itself by saying, "Costs have also risen for the best of reasons: medicine's improved ability to help people."

The publication that gave the most impetus and sanction to promoters of managed care was the *New England Journal of Medicine* which published a number of articles that claimed to demonstrate superiority of Kaiser *Permanente* and managed care. In 1990, it advocated managed care saying a new emphasis on managed care plans would encourage more physicians to join groups and affiliate with HMOs, and that fee-for-service practice was a "luxury" that government and business could "no longer afford to subsidize."[25] In 1991, it got on the bandwagon of managed care saying, and was widely quoted, that managed care was indeed the solution to America's health care financing problem. By 1993, editors at the *New England Journal of Medicine* began to have reservations about the endorsement of managed care saying that most management of care was accomplished indirectly by insurance companies through the management of costs, and that encouraging price competition among insurers increased pressures on third parties to intrude into health care decisions.[26]

Was the evidence indeed overwhelming in favor of managed care? Had the *New England Journal of Medicine* been worn down by promoters of managed care? Enthusiasm for managed care swept through the nation's businesses, the

[25] A.S. Relman. "Reforming the Health Care System." *New England Journal of Medicine* 323 (1990) 991-992.
[26] A.S. Relman. "Controlling Costs by 'Managed Competition'—Would It Work?" *New England Journal of Medicine* 328 (1993) 133-135.

Congress, and the White House. No wonder it came to the same conclusion as the editors of *Medical Economics* and of business and management magazines, that managed care is "here to stay," although doctors in our community who had lived with Kaiser *Permanente* were disturbed by the unrealistic promotion of managed care by the press. By July 1995, the *New England Journal of Medicine* asserted that the rush toward managed care was "wrong headed"![27]

Popular magazines and professional journals gave a sanction to the promoters of managed care liken to venal journalism that occurs in the case of finance and banking manias and mass movements, such as touting of financial manias by financial writers and financial columnists. Columnists tend to support manias, not always responsibly, and only occasionally are they critical of financial and banking manias.[28] In 1898, Le Bon cautioned that the power of the daily press had grown immeasurably: "a power the more to be feared because it is without limit, without responsibility, without control, and is exercised by anonymous and absolute individuals."[29]

The men of words in the press, by a one-sided argument towards managed care, enlisted the frustrated, undermined established norms and institutions.

II. 6. RHETORIC OF MANAGED MEDICAL CARE

Managed care thrived on rhetoric; 'Embrace', the operative word in the rhetoric of managed care, means to take or clasp in the arms, press to the bosom, hug, etc. "Embrace" in managed care is more akin to 'embrace' in law, which means "to attempt to influence a judge or jury through corrupt means" (def. 2).[30] The public, medical profession and hospital administrators were admonished to "embrace" managed care in a mass appeal.

The phrase "managed care" itself implied the welfare of patients, but raised suspicion that care was managed to maximize income for employers, health plans, and stockholders while masquerading as a benefit for community health, or

---

[27] J. Kassirer. "Managed Care and the Morality of the Marketplace." *New England Journal of Medicine* 333 (1995) 50-52.
[28] Charles P. Kindleberger. *Manias, Panics, and Crashes: A History of Financial Crises.* Third Edition. New York, Chichester, Brisbane, Toronto, Singapore: John Wiley, 1996. p. 75.
[29] Gustave Le Bon. *Psychologie du Socialisme* or *The Psychology of Socialism*. Paris: F. Alcan, 1898. in Alice Widener. *Gustave Le Bon: The Man and His Works.* Indianapolis: Liberty Press, 1979. p. 125.
[30] *The Random House Dictionary of the English Language.* Unabridged, 1966.

managing costs in preference to managing care.[31] The term "managed care" was inapt since 'care' requires flexibility and judgment, whereas 'managed' implies rigidity and rules.[32]

Rhetoric of managed care exhibited similarities, if not the same motives, as quackery of the nineteenth century. Throughout most of the history of Western society, medicine shows reaped a golden harvest for charlatans with nostrums and fake remedies advertised with high-pressure techniques. Brazen and suave, quacks persuaded the credulous to part with their money in exchange for a false hope, with the promises "infallible," "speedy," and "permanent."

Although the movement flourished during the nineteenth century, it extended well into the mid-twentieth century in the person of Dr. John R. Brinkley who made a fortune, not by his medical skill, but by the most modern of managed care techniques: his genius lay in marketing and advertising. The rhetoric of managed care and of quackery, whether in past centuries or the present, are the same—preying on the gullible. Medical advertising was held in disrepute and denounced as unethical until recently when advertising, not so much by physicians, but by hospitals, insurance companies, and managed care plans saturated the media. The slogans were remarkably similar to those of today:

'Preferred Provider' implied that physicians were selected on basis of merit, when in fact, 'preferred' amounted to the willingness of doctors to take substantially reduced fees to protect the viability and profits of health care plans.

The slogan 'health maintenance organization,' far removed from any sort of maintenance of health activity, existed as a distorted name for capitation and profit, *An Imposter Term.*

Does *'Permanente'* promise or imply permanence? or everlasting good health? eternal youth?

The use of slogans pushed with brazen and unscrupulous language by managed care companies, and other health promoters as cure-alls, panaceas, and specifics fueled the mass movement towards managed care. Rather than phony hustlers, these purveyors were suave and pricey consultants—a new generation of 'toadstool millionaires.' Even the phrase "health care" derogates the tradition of the medical profession. A "vertically integrated" hospital system called the *New York Hospital for the Ruptured and the Lame* would not survive under managed care rhetoric because it advertises expertise for those who might seek care.

---

[31] John H. McArthur and Francis D. Moore. "The Two Cultures and the Health Care Revolution: Commerce and Professionalism." *Journal of the American Medical Association* 277 (1997) 985-989.

[32] Fred Rosner. "Managed Care: Ethical Issues." Letter. *Journal of the American Medical Association* 274 (1995) 609-610.

Although high-pressure tactics of quacks of the nineteenth century seem comical, high-pressure nostrum peddlers of the managed care industry of today are their equals: "infallible," "speedy," and "permanent(e)." Metaphors, clichés, buzzwords, and slogans were synonymous with managed care, bringing with it a mass of meaningless words and shibboleths. Here are more that require little explanation:

"Incentive" equated to action is probably the most cited error of managed care, especially by economists and health care consultants, the *Fallacy of Equivocation* or confusing two literal meanings of a word.

"Reform" necessitates a crisis for its currency—error of *petitio principii* begs the question.

Physicians and patients came to feel that they were captives of the managed care industry; that they were owned by health plans: "They have us. There is no fighting it."

As in the case of banking manias, managed care especially called into play meteorological metaphors: the oppressive atmosphere that precede storms, earthquakes, or a presentiment of disaster.[33] Managed care is likened to: "Gathering storm clouds!" "Black, boiling clouds!" And:

- Crisis: "What went wrong?" "Skyrocketing medical costs." "Bloated costs."
- Fear: "Revenue lock-out" "Attributes of survival." "Incredible market forces."
- Appeal to emotion: "Traveling down the steep slope of managed care." "When is revolution coming? It is already here!"
- Greed: "Payors pushing rich contracts at you." "No longer hospital admissions, but capitated lives." "Look at what is happening in hot markets."
- Mania: "We've got to make this thing work!" "Re-inventing health care all over again."
- "It doesn't count if you can't count it," an often-repeated slogan of the managed care industry, exhibits the fallacy of *argumentum ad ignorantiam*: what isn't known to be true is false.

---

[33] Charles P. Kindleberger. *Manias, Panics, and Crashes: A History of Financial Crises.* Third Edition. New York, Chichester, Brisbane, Toronto, Singapore: John Wiley, 1996, p. 86.

Freud noted the remarkable power of words, that reason and arguments are incapable of combating certain words and formulas, and that an individual in a group is no longer an individual, but becomes an automaton who ceases to be guided by his will.[34] Words persuade individuals, by rhetoric and emotion, that managed care was a revolution, and that it was impossible to resist. Fear of medicine, probably based in a fear of illness and tragedy, leads to illogical decisions, including the rush towards managed care. As in the case of quackery, advertising became increasingly sophisticated, sometimes composed by MDs and PhDs, making pseudoscience sound like science.

That the practice of fee-for-service medicine was "admittedly flawed," or "deeply flawed," that only by lowering the profession of medicine—doctors and hospitals—can bring a beneficial change was recited by a profusion of consultants and critics of medicine permitted the managed care industry to flourish. In that no human endeavor has ever been without flaw, the assertion that any style of medical financing is "flawed" lacks meaning but worked as effective propaganda. By declaring a "crisis," rhetoric of mass movement into managed care corresponds to passionate, exaggerated claims, leading to excitement and embracing the movement.

Mass movements put an almost unlimited trust in language believing that if language is used appropriately it can persuade men to believe what the mass believes, and do what the mass wants them to do. Grammar of persuasion is based on affirmation and repetition, its two sovereign rules. The basic condition for any propaganda is to put forward a unilateral position or a dominant idea, clearly presented in a way that allows no retort. Its content of information may be slender, and does not need to contain anything that those hearing it do not already know.[35]

If promising to contain solutions to all problems, the most ill defined words and slogans possess the greatest influence. Words uttered with solemnity in presence of crowds, as soon as they have been pronounced, an expression of respect is visible on every face, and heads bow. Words make grandiose and vague images in men's minds, but this vagueness that wraps them in obscurity augments their mysterious power. The only figure of rhetoric of serious importance—repetition—forms a "current of opinion" leading to contagion and imitation. In time, ideas propagated by affirmation, repetition, and contagion acquire the mysterious force of *prestige*—a domination exercised by an individual, a work, or

[34] Max Hernandez. Group Formation and Ideology. Text and Context." *International Journal of Psycho-Analysis* 69 (1988) 163-170.
[35] Serge Moscovici. *The Age of the Crowd: A Historical Treatise on Mass Psychology*. Translated by J.C. Whitehouse. Cambridge, London, and New York: Cambridge University Press, 1985, pp. 144-145.

an idea. Prestige paralyses critical faculty, and "fills our soul with astonishment and respect," the mainspring of all authority.[36]

Propaganda is more fervent when in conjunction with coercion, such that propaganda serves to justify to oneself more than to convince others, and tends to relieve guilt. Coercion by the true believer not only subdues the opponent, but also intensifies his own faith in the movement. The coerced convert to a mass movement like managed care tends to be as fanatic as the persuaded convert, and sometimes more so. Coercion has an unequaled persuasiveness, not only with simple people but also with people of strength and integrity of intellect. Conquest and conversion go hand in hand, conversion justifying conquest.[37]

II. 7. FEAR

Fear suppressed resistance adding momentum to the managed care industry by creating alarm among doctors, hospitals, and the public. Fear suppressed rebellion with predictions of doom keeping doctors, hospitals and patients on the edge of personal and collective doubt. The cause for fear was real—not merely in concept: doctors were quitting practice, giving up and joining staff-model HMOs like Kaiser *Permanente*, or leaving medicine. Warnings and cautions by medical liability insurance companies on tactics of the managed care industry took their toll. Managed care shifted responsibility and liability from the medical insurance industry to doctors and other providers.

Price competition for contracts among health care providers was the primary *modus operandi* of the managed care industry. Fear became a major force of change among health care providers and was particularly influential. Physicians who found themselves in an insecure position as "oversupplied resources" were asked by managed care companies to change their practices. Yet, to blame physicians for the rise in medical care costs was like blaming the police for crime.

As doctors were set against each other, the psychic toll on physicians became immense with our sense of community and collegiality torn apart: how quickly the astonishing became commonplace.[38] Fear leads to defensiveness and cover-ups, rather than to honest, open searching for problems and ways of correcting them. The managed care industry was little interested in the ethics or morality of

---

[36] Gustave Le Bon. *The Crowd: A Study of the Popular Mind.* (1925) Dunwoody, GA: Norman S. Berg, 2nd ed. 1984. pp. 96-97, 127.

[37] Hoffer. pp. 98-100.

[38] Philip R. Alper. "Medical Practice in the Competitive Market." *New England Journal of Medicine* 316 (1987) 337-339.

physicians because physicians were not judged by managed care plans or improvement of their patients' health, nor were physicians evaluated to see if they were delivering adequate care. More than a failure of concept, medical practices and clinics failed, and even established staff-model HMOs failed, while health care consultants said that fear was a better motivator than greed.[39]

Fear was also a major force in the decisions of patients. The demand for health care "reform" did not rest in the 15% of Americans who, from time to time, were uninsured, or even from the smaller percentage who were hard-core uninsured; rather, fear came from the 85% of the people of this country who had health insurance and were fearful that they were going to lose it.[40] According to Mark Twain, "The fear of not knowing makes first class illnesses out of second-rate problems."

Fear and suspicion become the rule in a mass movement. Innocent people are deliberately accused and sacrificed in order to keep fear and suspicion alive. Opposition from within the mass threatens the movement by claims of association with the opposition from without. This enemy—the indispensable devil (fee-for-service medical practice)—is omnipresent who plots both outside and inside the mass, whose voice speaks through the dissenter. If anything goes wrong within the movement, it is the dissenter's doing. The true believer in the mass movement of managed care must be suspicious, to be constantly on the lookout for nonconformists by utilization review committees and by review clerks in managed care plans' corporate offices. Mutual suspicion within the mass is compatible with both its collective strength and a precondition of it. Mutual suspicion connects them with a mutual dread, binds them together, prevents desertion, and braces them for moments of weakness.[41]

The managed care industry traded on the insecurities and fears of the public, the hospitals, and those in the profession of medicine. Fear hastened mania of the managed care mass movement.

[39] Joseph M. Davis. "Predicting Future Health System Change" *Health Affairs* Winter 15 (1996) 107-108.
[40] Hon. Howard Dean. "The States as Health Reform Laboratories." in *Beyond the Crisis: Preserving the Capacity for Excellence in Health Care and Medical Science* Henry M. Greenberg and Susan U. Raymond, editors. *Annals of the New York Academy of Sciences* 729 (1994) 91-94.
[41] Hoffer. pp. 114-115.

Chapter III

ENTHUSIASM. CONTAGION

III. 1. SUPPORTIVE DATA TURN UP

A mass movement like managed care must develop supportive data. A new model is not brought about by discovery of new facts. Creation of demand for a new model to suit particular needs can be produced almost at will, which reflects prevalent psychology as much as it reflects the state of knowledge. The old is not demolished by an on-rush of new phenomena; new supportive data obediently turn up. The new model of managed care need not make objective sense, because data can be made to fit. The new will not be set up without evidence; evidence will turn up when need becomes sufficiently great. It may be true evidence, since evidence received occurs in response to questions asked.[1]

Concepts that make the foundation of managed care may actually be 'real' data, that is, gathered, statistically analyzed and pronounced valid. Studies funded by managed care industry tended to turn out in a way that supported the mass movement of managed care. Data supportive to the notion of managed care, however, persisted even after evidence has been disproved and refuted by experience. In this case, the data are not part of hankering for a new model, but a manipulation of the public mind in form of propaganda, eventually risking denial of contrary data, or *anchoring*.

Propagandists focus on target groups by age, intelligence and education to gain attention, especially by repetition such that distortions become inevitable with a goal of eliminating all competition. Propaganda techniques of name

---

[1] C.S. Lewis. *The Discarded Image: An Introduction to Medieval and Renaissance Literature.* Cambridge, Cambridge University Press, 1964, p. 223.

calling, glittering generalities, transfer or borrowing symbols with strong value for use in a new way, testimonials from persons with prestige, "plain folks," card stacking, selection, distorting or falsifying facts, led to the bandwagon effect of managed care.[2]

Supportive data must turn up at the beginning of the movement whether real or contrived by advocating a "mysterious absurdity" for the movement to gain momentum. At certain times, frustration may be so intense that almost any proselytizing mass movement finds the situation ready-made for its propagation.[3]

III. 2. BASIC CONCEPTS OF MANAGED CARE

The underlying concepts that led to adoption of managed care are neither new, innovative, nor experimental. Since the managed care industry is over a half-century old, it no longer holds promise of a splendid, glorious future. Kaiser *Permanente* and the managed care industry based its medical practice on a simplistic, production-model or assembly-line concept of delivering medical care: primary care was good enough—expertise was not needed, or at least not needed very often because specialty care was deemed expensive.

Assumptions of the pre-paid plan that became Kaiser *Permanente* were:

- Vast sums could be saved by elimination of waste, inefficiency, and duplication it claimed were prevalent in hospitals by an assembly-line type of medical practice, but not to the extent that those at Kaiser *Permanente* expected, nor was Kaiser *Permanente* able to eliminate these conditions from their own facilities.
- Assembly-line medicine caused many dissatisfactions and problems and was soon de-emphasized.
- The general public was not sophisticated enough to know good medical care from bad medical care: that it was not necessary to provide the best, or the most desirable medical care.

On assumption that providing medical care was simple and uncomplicated, a simplistic assembly-line plan for providing medical care was claimed to separate the "well," "worried-well," "early-sick" and "sick" into clear-cut groups by use of

---

[2] S. Stanfeld Sargent and Robert C. Williamson. *Social Psychology: An Introduction to the Study of Human Relations*. New York: The Ronald Press, 1958, pp. 449-450.
[3] Eric Hoffer. *The True Believer*. New York: Harper & Row, 1951, p. 114.

medical technology and computers operated by non-physician personnel.[4] The result was a mass of data that no one could interpret and did not lead to cost savings. Cynicism became the operative mode of the managed care industry fashioned after its paradigm of Kaiser *Permanente*. The concept of managed care was based on cost control by:

- Prevention.
- Primary, pre-hospital care.
- Limited access to hospitals and specialty care.
- Competition (see III. 7).

Over the course of five decades, managed care was promoted on a number of additional concepts: ideas purported to reduce costs of care, maintain or enhance quality of medical care, and to justify the growth and sanction of managed care at the expense of regular fee-for-service practice. The principal claims are considered below. Each concept has been evaluated: none are new or innovative, and all have failed to reduce over-all costs.

Prevention

That prevention, the cornerstone of managed care promotion, lowers health care costs seemed self-evident: prevention of illnesses must surely reduce medical costs. So insistent were claims about prevention one might think the managed care industry invented preventive medicine. Prevention has been a basic principle of medical practice for millennia, and preventive medicine one of great achievements of the nineteenth century.

As early as 1970, prevention was championed as the principal method of controlling health care costs, and that "incentives" of 'health maintenance organizations' would lead towards preventive medicine, primary care before inpatient care was needed, and to do everything possible to keep or make their members healthy. Rhetoric of prevention to officials of HEW was called "inspirational" and "evangelical" such that "revelation" replaced "disbelief."[5]

So pervasive was the notion of prevention's role in controlling health care costs that managed care companies placed extraordinary emphasis on it with claims of "unique Wellness Programs that give the managed care company a

---

[4] Sidney Garfield. "The Delivery of Medical Care." *Scientific American* 222 (1970) 15-23.

marketing advantage over its competitors."[6] Medical school professors also adopted the inherent good of prevention in lower health care costs. Advocates of managed care declared that HMOs had an incentive to keep elderly enrollees healthy in order to reduce managed care company costs.[7] In Medicare managed care companies, greatest profits were expected to come from keeping hospitalization days down by "keeping seniors healthy."[8]

Prevention in managed care ended with marketing. Claims of "wellness" appealed to members in consumer surveys, even though most managed care plans had no health-risk reduction programs whatsoever.[9]

Preventive practices for healthy living are indeed associated with better health and longer lives. Changes in lifestyle were proposed for everyone, as though everyone was at equal risk, however, lifestyle changes carry risks.[10] "Prevention saves money" was persistently stated in repetitive, hypnotic managed care propaganda. Although preventive care is good for health, prevention does *not* save money. Even in those few instances where prevention may save on costs, managed care plans had little motivation to act because patients tended to change managed care plans every few years. With investor profits in mind, preventive care that might save money in ten years became less attractive to managed care plans, especially if prevention costs would become a benefit after patients changed to another managed care plan. Prevention was parlayed into marketing propaganda, little more than a colored brochure.

Some diseases that have been remarkably controlled through preventive medicine are: small pox, typhus fever, typhoid fever, cholera, yellow fever, the plague, tuberculosis, diphtheria, pneumonia, rabies, malaria, venereal diseases, leprosy, and puerperal or child-bed fever—all long before the arrival of managed care.[11]

Preventing diseases involves risks as well as benefits although risks are usually low. Even when the financial cost of the preventive measure looks small, full costs are often larger than savings. A clearly low risk for prevention does not mean that prevention is preferable, since more people are subject to a prevention

[5] Lawrence D. Brown. *Politics and Health Care Organization: HMOs as Federal Policy.* Washington, DC: The Brookings Institution, 1983, pp. 206-207.
[6] *Form 10-K Annual Report*: Year Ending Dec 31, 1996: Health Systems International, Inc.
[7] Ken Terry. "You can thrive under managed care." *Medical Economics* April 7 (1997) 12-25.
[8] Deborah A. Grandinetti. "What it takes for big groups to succeed." *Medical Economics* April 7 (1997) 87-98.
[9] Michael A. Hiltzik and David Olmos. "Do HMOs Ration Their Health Care?" *Los Angeles Times.* August 27, 1995.
[10] Louise B. Russell. *Is Prevention Better Than Cure?* Washington, DC: The Brookings Institution, 1986, p. 106.
[11] Russell. p. 1.

measure than to the disease, and people who suffer from a preventive measure may not be the same as ones who would have suffered from the disease, which becomes more important the more uncertain estimates of risk.[12]

Unlike vaccination, screening alone has no direct health benefit—screening identifies people who may benefit from treatment. Evaluation of a screening test must consider not only risks of a disease, but those of the test itself. Often risks of prevention cannot be fully understood until a preventive measure has been applied to large populations for a long time.[13] Most screening tests must be repeated at regular intervals, and even in case of some cancers, with improvement in treatment, importance of screening tests diminishes.[14]

Prevention does not lead to lower medical expenditures as well as better health. By insisting on both, proponents of prevention as a way of lowering health care costs put themselves in the untenable position of arguing that a preventive measure is a good investment only if it saves money. Only a rare preventive measure, like smallpox vaccine, eradicates the condition altogether; anti-hypertensive drugs and regular exercise, for example, reduce occurrence of but do not eliminate heart attacks. Acute care remains necessary for those who suffer the disease despite reasonable efforts to prevent it.[15]

During the past century, preventive medicine revolutionized how most Americans lived. Immunizations, cleaner air and food, improved water and sewage systems, safer home and work environments, nutrition, and regular exercise protected populations from infection and injury. As a direct result, leading causes of death in the US are now those that most often come with age. Even these pose less of a threat due to improved diagnostic tests, medications, and surgery. Nevertheless, political campaigns during the 1990s claimed that increased prevention would cut medical spending. Yet, in studies of disease prevention measures, only three paid for themselves: prenatal care for poor women, tests in newborns for some congenital disorders, and some childhood immunizations. Prevention of *all* diseases would result in an aging population undergoing biological decay, which would live longer and cost more while they were dying.[16]

By advertising wellness and prevention, managed care companies attracted a lower risk population.[17] Despite emphasis placed on prevention by the managed

---

[12] Russell. pp. 3, 8.

[13] Russell. pp. 76, 78, 110.

[14] Kristin Leutwyler. "The Price of Prevention." *Scientific American* Apr 1995; Elisabeth Rosenthal. "When Healthier Isn't Cheaper: The HMO Catch." *New York Times* March 16, 1997.

[15] Russell. pp. 111-112.

[16] Leutwyler.

[17] Leutwyler.

care industry, even after allowing for savings in treatment, prevention adds to medical expenditures, contrary to the popular view that it reduces costs.[18]

The illusion of eternal youth, or the promise of perfect health by means of advertising prevention, the managed care industry preyed on the gullible, a phenomenon which has survived over millennia: "If pursuing disadvantage after the disadvantage has become obvious is irrational, then rejection of reason is the prime characteristic of folly."[19]

Primary Care with Limited Access to Specialty Care

Health maintenance organizations embraced *primary care* to promote health, prevent illnesses, diagnose early onset of disease, and manage all patient-encounters within the health care system. However, specialization furthers the cause of general education, and general medicine. Specialization became an inevitable aspect of progress, medical knowledge, and greater productivity.

Although general internal medicine physicians and primary care doctors were given top place in the scheme of managed care, patients tended to move from primary care doctor to primary care doctor on changes of their company's managed care plans. A cardiologist noted that many of his patients had a new primary doctor each year, such that specialists provided continuity of care instead of primary care physicians.[20] Board certification in primary care does not confer extensive knowledge needed to manage complex diseases, many of which have been identified in the past twenty years.[21] For example, patients with myocardial infarction, or heart attacks, treated by specialists in cardiology were treated more efficiently with better outcomes, shorter length of hospital stay, and achieved a lower mortality than those treated by family doctors or doctors of internal medicine.[22]

In numerous rheumatic disorders, early appropriate intervention can reduce morbidity, maintain function, and prolong life. Timely treatment improves outcome, reduces costs, or both. Regular care by a rheumatologist achieves better

---

[18] Russell. p. vii.

[19] Barbara W. Tuchman. *The March of Folly: From Troy to Vietnam*. New York: Ballatine, 1984, p. 380.

[20] Philip R. Alper. "Managed care, too, shall pass-the sooner the better." *Medical Economics* 17 June (1991) 93-96.

[21] Lonny Reisman. "It's the *Medicine*, Stupid." in *Beyond the Crisis: Preserving the Capacity for Excellence in Health Care and Medical Science* Henry M. Greenberg and Susan U. Raymond, editors. *Annals of the New York Academy of Sciences* 729, 1994, pp. 186-187.

mobility and function in patients with rheumatoid arthritis in comparison with intermittent care. Restricted access to specialists was based on the assumption that specialists were more costly, less controllable, and sometimes unnecessary in comparison to primary care physicians. Evidence that these beliefs were true in any instance, or true for *all* specialties, was sparse. Reduced utilization of services for elderly patients with joint pain was observed in health maintenance organizations with Medicare risk contracts; these patients had poorer outcomes than patients not enrolled in managed care plans.[23]

In the early days of Kaiser *Permanente*, the "multi-phasic" *annual examination* was acclaimed to maintain good health and to establish a baseline of health status. The "multi-phasic" examination consisted of a number of tests that could be easily automated and performed inexpensively, such as automatic blood counts and chemistry tests, a three inch chest X-ray, and a two lead electrocardiogram, which was followed by an office visit with a physician or nurse practitioner. Although no cost savings were realized, the multi-phasic examination was heavily promoted to the point that once begun, the practice could not be stopped without Kaiser *Permanente* losing appearances.

During early 1970s, Kaiser *Permanente* itself discovered that *early detection* of health problems and early treatment did not reduce over-all costs. Outcomes of many medical conditions could not be altered as expected and required continued care. Costs of surveillance of a large population to find few medical conditions that were actually remediable by early diagnosis and treatment far exceeded costs of treatment. Identifying illnesses at an early stage led to a longer period of observation and treatment, and *greater*—not lesser—costs.[24]

The *gatekeeper*, or primary physician, had responsibility to authorize tests or referrals to specialists. Capitation-plus-bonus financial arrangements turned gatekeepers into gateshutters undermining trust between physician and patient.[25] Belatedly, the gatekeeper model proved to be expensive, wasteful, and a failed notion. Gatekeepers resided in offices of managed care health plans with treatment guidelines on a computer. Computer-based technologies when given a

---

[22] J. Duncan Moore, Jr. "Special Treatment: Study compares results by different kinds of doc." *Modern Healthcare* Mar 17 (1997) 17.

[23] Committee of the American College of Rheumatology on Health Care Research. "Role of Specialty Care for Chronic Disease: Ad Hoc Committee of the American College of Rheumatology." *Mayo Clinic Proceedings* 71 (1996) 1179-1181.

[24] Gary D. Friedman, Marshall Goldberg, Jagan N. Ahuja, A.B. Siegelaub, Milton L. Bassis, and Morris I. Cohen. "Biochemical Screening Tests: Effect of Panel Size on Medical Care." *Arch Internal Medicine* 129 (1972) 91-97; *Medical Tribune*, Thursday, August 28, 1969. cited in "Multiphasic Data Gives Labs Problems." *ACCMA Bulletin*, vol. 25. Nov. 1969, p. 37.

[25] Thomas Bodenheimer. "The HMO Backlash—Righteous or Reactionary?" *New England Journal of Medicine* 335 (1996) 1601-1604.

case history may be able to access guidelines and identify appropriate care in a particular case 80 percent of the time, leaving 20 percent of problems incorrectly identified.[26]

The gatekeeper idea of managed care failed. Eventually, health plans approved the vast majority of specialty referrals, so that gatekeepers didn't save money, and gatekeepers could be surmounted by a persistent patient or persistent doctor.[27] Moreover, obstacles to specialty care might very well harm patients and heighten liability risk for physicians and health plans, and increase insurance costs. Since 99 percent of tests and treatments were eventually authorized, savings gained by a gatekeeper, if any, was offset by administrative costs of gatekeeping, often over trivial items, as well as time consuming nuisance factor. Primary physicians assumed a responsibility and liability for which they were rarely paid or paid adequately: physician, front-office and back-office workload increased dramatically without reimbursement to cover added expenses. Gatekeeping was a way for managed care plans to squeeze more and more from providers.

Lower Rates of Surgery

In late 1970s, rate or frequency of surgery at Kaiser *Permanente* was claimed to be 19.6 percent lower than in comparable population in regular fee-for-service practice, and some claimed as much as a 30% lower rate of surgery in some managed care plans. The implication of impropriety of the regular fee-for-service physicians—an excessive number of surgical procedures—seemed obvious and promoted claims against fee-for-service physicians and surgeons emphasized in the press. Kaiser *Permanente* and the managed care industry accepted the claims without complaint and capitalized on it. Blue Cross, with a vested interest in finding as many examples of unnecessary surgery as possible to apply pressure on fee-for-service doctors, examined 2,275 consecutive surgical cases expecting to find 400 to 600 unnecessary surgical cases, and found, not the 19.6 percent to 30 percent of unnecessary cases, but 0.6 percent of cases that were considered unnecessary, which nullified one of the most insistent claims of advocates of managed care. The implication that treatment was denied by Kaiser *Permanente* or that a selected population accounted for the difference did not appear in the press. The silence of those at Kaiser *Permanente* and those promoting managed

---

[26] Mark Holoweiko. "Bypassing primary-care physicians." *Medical Economics* Apr 14 (1997) 208-219.

[27] George Anders. *Health Against Wealth: HMOs and the Breakdown of Medical Trust.* Boston and New York: Houghton Mifflin, 1996, p. 245.

care was astonishing. In addition, Blue Cross-Blue Shield of Greater New York abandoned second opinions of elective surgery long ago because nearly all of recommended surgery was found to be reasonably indicated by original surgeons further emphasizing distortion of claims about alleged unnecessary surgery in fee-for-service practice of medicine.[28]

Additional concepts of managed medical care that have failed to reduce costs[29]:

- Lower rates of hospitalization.
- Lower cost of hospitalization.
- Shorter hospital stays.
- Outpatient therapy and home care.
- Group practice or vertical integration.
- Centralization of services, or consolidation of facilities.
- Economies of scale.
- Reduced emergency room usage.
- Practice profiles and practice guidelines.
- Claims of better outcomes.
- Care of chronic illness and the elderly.
- Comprehensive, broad coverage.
- Accountability and oversight of care.
- Limiting or rationing care.
- Efficiency.
- Electronic medical record.
- Sick call, or drop-in practice.
- The use of midwives instead of obstetricians.
- The use of nurse practitioners instead of physicians.
- Mandatory arbitration.
- Computerized medical record.

Although basic concepts of managed care failed to reduce costs, the rush towards managed care proceeded without restraint in *believe perserverance* and *confirmatory bias*, or "wooden-headedness," the source of self-deception in assessing a situation in preconceived, fixed notions while ignoring or rejecting

---

[28] *ACCMA Bulletin* Feb. 1981, p. 8.
[29] R.D. Smith. *Managed Care: Anatomy of a Mass Medical Movement.* The Rhodes-Fulbright Library, Bristol, IN: Wyndham Hall Press, 2000, 69-98.

contrary signs. Wooden-headedness, acting according to wish while not allowing oneself to be deflected by facts, plays a remarkably large role in government and human affairs,[30] such as promotion of the mass movement of managed care.

III. 3. MEDICAL TECHNOLOGY

Development and widespread application of medical technology received much of the responsibility for increased health care costs. Some argued that because a new technology was available that doctors use it at every possible occasion regardless of its usefulness. According to managed care proponents, if an incentive to over-utilize technology existed, then technology was over-utilized at every possible opportunity because technology is "demand enhancing"—an argument from the particular to the general, that if a few doctors over-use technologies, all are guilty of the offense.

Never in history has the medical profession been presented with so many powerful new technologies, new methods of treatment, and new effective medicines, such as the CT scanner, which produces remarkable images heretofore unavailable except at surgery or at autopsy. Hemodialysis, total joint replacements, cardiac pacemakers, cataract lens implants are examples of new technological advances with enormous humanitarian, social and economic impact. The United States is ahead of other countries in that most new technologies are developed and produced here, and are relatively inexpensive and widely available. During the late 1940s and 1950s, the most important technologic advance in medicine, antibiotic drugs, sharply reduced the average length of hospital stays, which should warn against blanket indictment of technology as "cost-enhancing."[31]

Such a profusion of technological advances wasn't a dream a half century ago when managed care industry had its beginning. Not just new technology, but technologies that work, that save lives, relieve suffering, cure some diseases and meliorate many others. Refinements and improvements will continue, but many of the major areas of opportunity for technological advancement have been met. "Breakthrough" became a household word for the marvels of science-based medicine. It is unlikely that such an era of innovation will occur again soon, while others say we are on the threshold of phenomenal new medical advances.

---

[30] Barbara W. Tuchman. p. 7; Matthew Rabin. "Psychology and Economics." *Journal of Economic Literature* 36 (1998) 11-46.

Lost in the managed care industry's rhetoric against paying for new advanced technologies, some technologies reduce health care costs. A quiet revolution occurred within the last decade in the management of one of medicine's greatest challenges: diabetes—especially insulin-dependent diabetes with the development of the home glucose meter.

After World War II, scientists developed new techniques to study human biochemistry leading to understanding of disease processes, which produced new anti-inflammatory drugs, anti-hypertension agents, and many others. An understanding of cell biology led to the development cancer chemotherapy and anti-viral agents. Biological technology produced recombinant DNA technology, monoclonal antibodies, and cell fusion techniques, as well as new drug delivery mechanisms. Nearly half of all world-class drugs developed between 1975 and 1989 originated in the US, more than three times the number developed in any other country.[32] Re-evaluation of medical treatments occurs constantly; accepted medical practices evolve and those found to be less effective than newer ones are supplanted as better therapies develop, that is, norm-oriented change.

Managed care contributed nothing to the development of new technologies, in fact, managed care with its regressive stance inhibited development of new and useful medical procedures and treatments by non-support of medical research and education. No technological advance can be attributed to the managed care industry.

III. 4. INTELLECTUAL UNDERPINNINGS

Principle arguments of the "health maintenance strategy" advocated by the Department of Health, Education and Welfare under Secretary Elliot Richardson were pressed forward by "promotional zeal" of Dr. Paul Ellwood.[33] The writings of Ellwood (1971), called "A 'visionary' who helped spur the nation's medical health care system into managed care,"[34] contain affect-laden rhetoric in emotive words: "much proclaimed health care crisis," "merely" providing care during

---

[31] Victor R. Fuchs. "The Health Sector's Share of the Gross National Product." *Science* 247 (1990) 534-538.

[32] Eran Broshy. "The Contribution of Pharmaceutical Companies: What's at Stake for America." in *Beyond the Crisis: Preserving the Capacity for Excellence in Health Care and Medical Science* Henry M. Greenberg and Susan U. Raymond, editors. *Annals of the New York Academy o f Sciences* 729, 1994. pp 118-123.

[33] Lawrence D. Brown. *Politics and Health Care Organization: HMOs as Federal Policy.* Washington, DC: The Brookings Institution, 1983. p. 211.

[34] Paul M. Ellwood. *Modern Healthcare* 13 Jan. (1989) 30-31.

illness, "fundamental reform," etc.[35] The leading fallacies, logical errors in the article's seven and a half pages are:

Glittering generalities	20
Imputation of bad design	18
Self-contradiction	12
Emotion-laden or emotive words	11
Erroneous statements, false claims	9
Argumentum ad imaginationem, appeal to fancy	8
Fallacy of distrust	8
Fallacy of pretended danger	8

In all, 192 errors in 41 categories of fallacies and errors of logic, bias, distortions, opinion, and slogans that appeal to emotion rather than reason.

The "intellectual underpinnings" of managed care would be expected to provide a sound and logical basis on which massive investment in resources would be justified, confidence that "intellectual underpinnings" can withstand rigorous challenge, that a wrenching change, a "one-hundred and eighty degree change" of medical practice into managed care, and that ethics, history and traditions of medicine can be justifiably discarded to "embrace" a new medical professional ethos.

An examination of the "intellectual underpinnings"[36] of managed care revealed a surprise: a logical structure based on false premises—a base of logical errors, fallacies, biased statements, speculation, grandiosity, magical thinking, and sham reasoning. Critics claimed that modern physicians were "cost unconscious" and out to fleece the public. By the error of *argumentum ad hominem* (collective, abusive), managed care advocates cried up managed care by crying down regular, fee-for-service practice of medicine.

From articles published by the venerable *New England Journal of Medicine* in 1978, an economist claimed that increases in health care spending "far exceeded what could be justified," the error of *converse accident* or hasty generalization, and that "[p]eople might be just as healthy with half as much

---

[35] Paul M. Ellwood, Jr., Nancy N. Anderson, James E. Billings, Rick J. Carlson, Earl J. Hoagberg, and Walter McClure. "Health Maintenance Strategy." *Medical Care* 9 (1971) 291-297.
[36] A.C. Enthoven and Sara J. Singer. "Managed Competition and California's Health Care Economy." *Health Affairs* Spring (1996) 40-57.

hospitalization,"[37] that is, speculation, *converse accident* or hasty generalization, an unsupported claim; and further claims that:

- "Fee-for-service has created a costly adversarial relationship between doctors and payers."
- "Fee-for-service has failed to create accountability for health outcomes and the outcomes information."
- "Fee-for-service 'free choice' leaves patients to make remarkably poorly informed choices of doctor."
- "Fee-for-service has left us with excess supply of specialists."
- "Fee-for-service has left us with major excesses in hospital beds, high-tech equipment, and open-heart surgery facilities."
- "[Fee-for-service has caused] a misallocation of resources."
- "Fee-for-service has led to a costly and dangerous proliferation in facilities for such complex procedures as open-heart surgery."
- "HMOs emphasize prevention, early diagnosis and treatment, and effective management of chronic conditions."[38]

Each statement above proved false. Yet, the mass movement of managed care sustained itself on authority of a consensus of self-styled experts: "The decisions affecting matters of general interest come to by an assembly of men of distinction, but specialists in different walks of life, are not sensibly superior to the decisions that would be adopted by a gathering imbeciles....In crowds it is stupidity and not mother-wit that is accumulated."[39] So frequent, relentless, and monotonous was the hypnotic tirade of logical errors and fallacies promoting managed care that they acquired an aura of truth, a prestige, to become part of the nation's mythic beliefs upon which it acted.

That HMOs achieve financial success by under-serving members, the same economist says, "I have been unable to find any documented case of a pattern of underservice among such HMO's,"[40] i.e. the error of *argumentum ad ignorantiam,* that what is not known to be true is false.

---

[37] A.C. Enthoven. "Consumer Choice Health Plan." *New England Journal of Medicine* 298 (1978) 650-658, 709-720.

[38] Enthoven and Singer (1996). A.C. Enthoven. "The History and Principles of Managed Competition." *Health Affairs* Supplement, 1993.

[39] Gustave Le Bon. *The Crowd: A Study of the Popular Mind.* Dunwoody, GA: Norman S. Berg, 2nd ed. 1984. p. 9.

[40] A.C. Enthoven. "Consumer Choice Health Plan." *New England Journal of Medicine* 298 (1978) 650-658, 709-720.

Mass movements do not arise until the prevailing order has been discredited, which is the deliberate work of fault-finding men and women-of-words with a grievance. Imperceptibly, the man-of-words undermines established institutions, discredits those in power, weakens prevailing beliefs and loyalties, and sets the stage for rise of a mass movement. The militant man-of-words prepares the masses for rise of a mass movement by subtle methods:

1. Discredits and detaches the allegiance of the people from prevailing creeds and institutions.
2. Indirectly creates a hunger for the movement, so that when the new idea is preached it finds an eager response among the mass.
3. Furnishes doctrine and slogans of the new movement.
4. Undermines convictions of the competent and secure—those who can get along without the mass movement—so that when a new fanaticism makes its appearance they are without capacity to resist.

The competent and secure see no sense in sacrificing for convictions and principles, and yield to the new order without a fight. The best lack all conviction, while the worst are full of passionate intensity.

Mass movements like managed care must have a devil, especially a devil with much good to its credit; managed care's devil was the regular fee-for-service practice of medicine by an appeal to enmity, by the School of Indictment, repeated often, relentlessly fostering an unstoppable mass movement. Its devil must be real, tangible, and accessible.

Mass movements become a throwback to a primitive society of collective existence where the individual has no importance. A mass movement emphasizes the present against the past, and the present considered mean in comparison to glories of the future. The present becomes a preliminary to the visions of the future and threshold of the millennium, as declared by some economists and advocates of managed care. Mass movements accentuate and perpetuate individual incompleteness of its adherents by elevating dogma above reason preventing individual intelligence from becoming self-reliant -- such that managed care enrollees surrendered individuality to lists of providers of managed care plans. The fault-finding man-of-words with a grievance persistently ridiculed and denounced prevailing beliefs and loyalties—not a society of freethinking individuals, but a corporate society that cherishes utmost unity and blind faith,[41]

---

[41] Hoffer. pp. 61-67, 119-127.

who set the stage for practical men and women-of-action, not men and women of ethics or morality, but of law, or what-can-be-gotten-away-with.

The "intellectual underpinnings" of the irrational mass movement of managed care form a *Noodle's Oration*: a superficially plausible argument consisting of fallacies and logical errors.[42]

III. 5. CONTRARY DATA

One of the principal features allowing spread of a mass movement and a popular delusion requires disregard of unwelcome news and contrary data. Only supportive opinions and reports are accepted, or if negative data are considered, it is to denounce them and suppress dissent; important cautions are not given appropriate weight. In 1978, serious limitations of managed care model were noted to be:

1. Time and cost to start.
2. To join, patients must change physicians, and managed care enrollment grew fastest among highly mobile populations, which periodically required people to find new physicians.
3. Perceived by patients as impersonal, institutional or inconvenient.
4. Unattractive to many physicians opposed to their professional independence.[43]

Financial incentives under managed care were known to be imperfect or that their performances were not without shortcomings. No logical or empirical basis existed for determining them *a priori*, and good incentives do not guarantee good performance. Medical care requires judgment and is fraught with uncertainty.[44] In California in 1978, examination of the mix of regular fee-for-service practice and managed care found "no evidence that even massive HMO enrollment had resulted in overall cost containment."[45]

[42] Sydney Smith. "Bentham on Fallacies" (1825), from the *Edinburgh Review*, in *The Works of the Rev. Sydney Smith*. New York: D Appleton and Co., 1864. pp. 218-219.
[43] A.C. Enthoven. "Shattuck Lecture—Cutting Cost Without Cutting Quality of Care." *New England Journal of Medicine* 298 (1978) 1229-1238.
[44] A.C. Enthoven. *Health Plan: the only practical solution to the soaring cost of medical care.* Addison-Wesley: Reading, Massachusetts, Menlo Park, California, 1980. p. 69.
[45] Harold S. Luft. "Health Maintenance Organizations, Competition, Cost Containment, and National Health Insurance." in Pauly, National Health Insurance, p. 304. cited by Lawrence D. Brown.

If we believe in the free market as an efficient and equitable mechanism for the distribution of most goods and services, many reasons caused worry about industrialization of health care: health care is different from commodities. To some degree, most people regard health care a basic right of all citizens: a public rather than a private good, and as a result, a large fraction of cost of medical research and medical care is subsidized by public funds. Classic laws of supply and demand do not operate in medical care because health-care consumers/patients do not have incentives to be prudent, discriminating purchasers, and never will. Heavy dependence of the consumer/patient on advice and judgment of physicians explains why economists' assumptions about a competitive free market do not apply to medical care who claimed that more than 70 percent of all expenditures for personal health are the result of decisions made by physicians. Goals of managed care and alleged wisdom of the marketplace were disputed; in an ideal free competitive market, private enterprise may be good at controlling unit costs, and even at improving quality of its products, but private businesses do not allocate their services or restrict use of them. On the contrary, they market their services and sell as many units as possible. Businesses may trim prices to sell more, but they are in business to increase total sales. Informed judgments of physicians acting in interest of their patients remain the best regulation of the health care marketplace.[46]

The Federal government chose to depend on market competition rather than regulation, but market forces have limited application and dubious ethical standing in health care. In any case, there was no evidence that competition was any more successful in keeping down costs than any other approach. The principal cause of the cost "crisis" was not so much price as increasing volume and intensity of medical services being provided. The managed care industry was expected to guarantee value *and* quality of services for patients at lower costs— not to generate the highest possible profits for the managed care industry. Without sufficient regulation, managed care escalated into a "medical arms race." In the San Francisco Bay Area, hospitals added more managers and marketing consultants to identify new 'product lines' and 'unmet community needs.'[47]

In the case of medical care, economic theory works only in fancy: medical costs were 26 percent higher for hospitals in highly competitive areas than in

Politics and Health Care Organization: HMOs as Federal Policy. Washington, DC: The Brookings Institution, 1983. p. 468.
[46] A.S. Relman. "The New Medical-Industrial Complex." *New England Journal of Medicine* 303 (1980) 963-970.
[47] Sypros Andreopoulos. "'Managed Competition' Is Health-Care Scam." Pacific News Service. 1992.

hospitals with no neighbors. The more competitors a hospital had the higher the costs. HMOs were supposed to have a "ripple effect" on others: in fact, costs were higher in competitive managed care markets. Calls for legislation to end insurance company discrimination against high-risk groups, such as those suffering from AIDS and chronic illnesses, went unheeded while an economist encouraged businesses to step up selection to avoid high utilization groups.[48]

Third-party management—managed care—increased hassles, substituted non-physician judgment, and spent an increasing share of medical resources on other than medical services. Managed care could not control costs, except by rationing.[49] The evidence about whether managed care plans saved money was unproved; managed care alone would not stem rising national health expenditures.[50]

The cry for "reform" at any cost and sanction of the managed care industry could not be rationally supported. Much that was blamed on the health care system resulted from social, educational, economic, or environmental problems: life-style accounts for 50% of factors affecting health of Americans, and the environment accounts for 20% which are not amenable to medical intervention or control, but reflect society's values and behavior. In addition, in 1991, 22% of health care costs were due to administrative costs that do not result in medical services.[51] Life expectancy in 1920 was 54 years, and in 1990 rose to 75 years, which entailed increased costs. Less than ten percent of increase in longevity over the past century was due to improvements in medical care, because socioeconomic status is the major determinate of health status. In countries where health care is "free," such as England, Switzerland, and Finland, poor health is closely linked to income level.[52]

Claims by promoters of managed care were impossible to substantiate: more and more studies showed favorable risk selection by managed care plan enrollees

---

[48] Andreopoulos. (1992).

[49] Joseph White. "Markets, Budgets, and Health Care Cost Control" *Health Affairs* Fall (1993) 44-57.

[50] John K. Iglehart. "Health Policy Report: The American Health Care System." *New England Journal of Medicine* 327 (1992) 742-747.

[51] George H. Kraft. "In Defense of Health Care: Preserving the Capacity for Excellence." in *Beyond the Crisis: Preserving the Capacity for Excellence in Health Care and Medical Science* Henry M. Greenberg and Susan U. Raymond, editors. *Annals of the New York Academy of Sciences* 729, (1994) 39-55.

[52] Cecil Pickett. "Impact of Health Care Reform on Research Innovativeness." in *Beyond the Crisis: Preserving the Capacity for Excellence in Health Care and Medical Science* Henry M. Greenberg and Susan U. Raymond, editors. *Annals of the New York Academy of Sciences* 729 (1994) 106-110.

relative to indemnity plans.[53] The General Accounting Office concluded that managed care plans cost more than fee-for-service plans. Medicare managed care plans had a greater proportion of healthy elderly so that managed care plans pocketed the difference in what was projected for the entire Medicare population. Managed care plans had an incentive to enroll those patients who were expected to have relatively low health-care costs. Medicare managed care plans discouraged enrollment by patients who were likely to need medical care, and once patients became ill, some managed care companies encouraged them to disenroll.[54] In Kaiser *Permanente* and the managed care industry, disastrous cases were written off as "anecdotal," a one-time, unusual occurrence that could have happened anywhere. Criticisms that were 'anecdotal' could be dismissed quickly, but anecdotes are evidence, and evidence accumulates to become general experience.[55]

The "near-worship" of primary care and exaggerated criticism of specialty care raised doubts that specialists are inherently too costly. Excessively critical fantasies about specialists coexisted with unduly flattering fantasies of primary-care physicians who were portrayed as paragons who could do nearly everything well. Claims of specialists' inefficiencies were written when the fashion was to leave no diagnostic stone unturned. Some specialists are the most cost-effective doctors for certain kinds of patients.[56]

Physicians were overwhelmed by accusations that we had been irresponsible in the matter of costs, that "double digit inflation" in health care costs could not be tolerated, and could not be sustained, that medical inflation was twice the general inflation. Yet, from 1971 to 1996, medical inflation hit double digits twice: 11.5% in 1975 and 10.5% in 1981. Twice during the same period, health care inflation was *below* the general inflation: 1973 and 1979.[57] Such data were not newsworthy to a venal press that encouraged the popular impression, which it helped to create, that fee-for-service practice was the cause of "runaway costs." As early as 1983, analysts knew that claims by the managed care industry were exaggerated if not false: evidence on relative effects of HMO and fee-for-service care on health

[53] Robert H. Miller and Harold Luft. "Managed Care Plan Performance Since 1980: A Literature Analysis." *Journal of the American Medical Association* 271 (1994) 1512-1519.

[54] John Merline. "Pay or Pay: Managed care will not save Medicare, but a dose of reality might." *National Review* 29 May 1995, p 45-48.

[55] Charles P. Kindleberger. *Manias, Panics, and Crashes.* 3rd ed. New York: John Wiley & Sons, 1996. p. 198.

[56] Philip R. Alper. "Specialists are getting a bum rap." *Medical Economics* 26 Feb 1996.

[57] *Internal Medicine News* March 15, 1997, page 1.

outcomes was equivocal and did not support that HMO care was better than fee-for-service care.[58]

Just as with banking manias, attempting to convince people of errors of their ways through talk is generally futile; contrary evidence about managed care was dismissed. When faced with complex and ambiguous evidence, the strength and reliability of confirming evidence is emphasized, but the weakness and unreliability of disconfirming evidence is overlooked. Indeed, ambiguities and conceptual flaws opposing their hypotheses may be regarded as somehow suggestive of the fundamental correctness of those hypotheses.[59] The true believer in a mass movement must close his eyes and ears to information that might abase faith in future of the mass movement. The infallibility of doctrine shields the believer from uncertainties, inconsistencies, and unpleasant realities around him. Strength of a mass movement depends on rejecting the present to center on the future, and it must make its adherents believe that it has already seen the future. The conflicts that a mass movement seeks and incites serve not only to down its enemies but also to strip its followers of their distinct individuality.[60]

In 1895, a social commentator said, "The masses have never thirsted after truth. They turn aside from evidence that is not to their taste, preferring to deify error, if error seduce them. Whoever can supply them with illusions is easily their master."[61] Contrary data had to be ignored for mass movement into managed care to expand.

III. 6. QUALITY

Quality of health care has been subjected to examination in one way or another since long before the days of Chaucer. In the early twentieth century, American medical schools were graded on overall quality, and all schools that were not Class A were closed. More recently, the matter of quality arose from the business community over the issue of costs. Many years of technological change were supported which improved quality of care but increased costs. Public expectations vastly increased while payers resisted,[62] which led to a search for measures of quality. Yet comparative information on quality between regular fee-for-service and managed care was lacking and little reliable information was

---

[58] Brown. p. 134.
[59] Kindleberger. p. 86; Rabin.
[60] Hoffer. pp. 76-78, 112.
[61] Le Bon. p. 190.
[62] Robert W. Hungate. "Whither Quality?" *Health Affairs* Winter 1996 111-113.

available on comparative quality of care in different hospitals and managed care companies.

Gathering measures of quality assessment was an expensive but important effort when health care competitors asserted their interest in "value," a combination of cost and quality. Some claimed that rigorous measures of quality were possible, but to implement them required money and time. A few inexpensive techniques have been used, but give only limited insight into a patient's medical condition, such as evidence about the relation of mortality rates and hospital quality was not clearly evident, with the risk of generating a mass of costly information but unable to determine its meaning.[63] No reliable method or level of analysis for performance measures are available that are useful to individual consumers.[64]

In absence of a reliable methodology that would give public and health plans objective data on quality, the managed care industry lacked a way of proving that its methods were desirable. Patient satisfaction surveys became the favored substitute even though surveys have a multitude of limitations. In any one year approximately 80% of covered population will not seek medical care with assured "satisfaction" making patient satisfaction surveys meaningless. Satisfaction surveys of those seeking care for serious illness may carry some validity, but none have been performed. Since morbidity and mortality are subject to manipulation by risk-avoidance of managed care health plans, these measures cannot be the principal criteria of effectiveness.[65]

Surveys can be even more misleading in that some of the best doctors would not score high in satisfaction surveys. These doctors take on the most difficult patients and the most difficult people. The most satisfied of individuals surveyed tend to be those most likely to respond to a survey questionnaire which distorts the actual number who are in fact satisfied. Nor is a favorable survey synonymous with medical skill or competence. Despite great effort and expenditure of resources, health plans and economists have been unable to measure quality of care with all of its current changes.[66] In addition, physicians participate in multiple health plans so that differentiating between managed care plans on basis of physician membership was impossible. Some have tried to develop 'decision

[63] Lisa Iezzoni. "How Much Are We Willing to Pay for Information about Quality?" *Annals of Internal Medicine* 126 (1997) 391-393.
[64] Gail L. Warden. "Chaotic, Shifting Relationships Of Purchasers, Plans, And Providers." *Health Affairs*. 15 Winter (1996) 116-117.
[65] John H. McArthur and Francis D. Moore. "The Two Cultures and the Health Care Revolution: Commerce and Professionalism." *Journal of the American Medical Association* 277 (1997) 985-989.
[66] Jack Lewin, John Muir Medical Center, Noon Conference 5-30-96.

analysis,' which attempted to formalize many things that experts do intuitively but often found difficult to explain.[67] That the practice of medicine is highly individual, a science-based art, creates barriers to objective and reliable measure of what physicians know intuitively.

Without trust, outcome-based medicine fails. If a patient or a family is to trust their physician's advice on futility of continued medical treatment, they must trust the physician. Numbers alone, even grim ones derived from thousands of cases and years of experience, will not suffice; and trust between physician and patient was jeopardized by the managed care mass movement.[68]

Regulation in an effort to give the appearance of quality was of little value in assessing the performance of the managed care industry. In California, the Department of Corporations regulated the managed care industry with its many plans and rapid changes. Many contended that the agency had not met minimal standards of enforcement. A former Department of Corporations investigator was quoted as saying that there is no regulation, "The Department of Corporations is doing nothing." Most methods attempting to measure quality are not measures of quality but measures of compliance. Compliance was mistaken for quality, the *fallacy of accent,* an invalid argument by a shift or change in meaning of words.

In the rush towards managed care, pursuit of quality played a minor role: the dominant motivation was lessening of expenditures. It was claimed that spending could be reduced in three ways:

1. Reducing services to patients.
2. Providing services more efficiently.
3. Reducing incomes of physicians and other health care providers.

Pressure on incomes of physicians and other health care suppliers does not create substantial gains for society as a whole; it is primarily a transfer of assets from one group to another.[69] Although managed care advocates claimed quality for their companies, quality was of little concern to the managed care industry; decisions were based on "price, price, price."[70] Whether we can assume that quality of medical care in managed care plans was comparable to that in fee-for-

---

[67] John K. Iglehart. "From Research to Rationing: A Conversation with William B. Schwartz." *Health Affairs* Fall 1989, 60-75.

[68] Arthur L. Caplan. "Odds and Ends: Trust and the Debate over Medical Futility." editorial. *Annals of Internal Medicine* 125 (1996) 688-689.

[69] Victor R. Fuchs. "Managed Care and Merger Mania." *Journal of the American Medical Association* 277 (1997) 920-921.

[70] Anders. (1996) p. 104.

service plans could not be demonstrated, or was managed care "next-best" treatment?[71] Or what-can-be-gotten-away-with treatment?

Those poorly served by HMOs have unusual or complex diseases that need specialized treatment or carefully coordinated care, and chronic conditions such as arthritis, multiple sclerosis, and stroke. Chronic diseases magnified all problems that existed for everyone in managed care. The process of getting authorization for treatment sometimes took months, and defied the claim of efficiency of the managed care industry. Patients with complicated or chronic illnesses found that rules to discourage overuse of medical resources functioned more as technicalities that could only be overcome by lengthy bureaucratic battles or court intervention.[72] 'Quality' as used in the managed care environment suggested "B- or C+ medical care," care that avoids immediate lethal consequences, an attempt to bring the bottom up to a very low acceptable mean; it represents "institutionalized mediocrity" and has nothing to do with excellence.[73] Doctors and patients could not accept that 'drive-through' deliveries and outpatient mastectomies were quality improvements, rather than cost-cutting measures. No proof developed as to whether managed care raised, lowered, or had no effect on quality. Market success of the managed care industry bore a weak link, if any, to quality of medical care.

Physicians have an interest in advertising excellence in order to do more of what they do well, and society has an interest in enabling patients with specific needs to go to physicians that excel at taking care of those needs. Managed care plans do not have mission statements that make them either interested or not interested in high-risk cases, but the financial consequences of enrolling difficult cases were clearly negative.[74]

Medicine has always been, and remains so today, an intensely personal relationship not readily testable for quality measures and remains an art. With managed care advocates' commitment of resources to pursuing the elusive nature of quality, to present something that satisfied an appearance of quality was essential in order to sustain the mass movement. Managed care promoters tried to develop and maintain the illusion of efficiency and quality, but managed care was the opposite. When a theory begins to fail, it is defended vigorously in attempts to 'save the appearances.' The illusion of quality was enough to satisfy business

[71] Hiltzik and Olmos. August 27, 1995.
[72] Hiltzik and Olmos. August 27, 1995.
[73] H.M. Greenberg. "Introduction." in *Beyond the Crisis: Preserving the Capacity for Excellence in Health Care and Medical Science* Henry M. Greenberg and Susan U. Raymond, editors. *Annals of the New York Academy of Sciences* 729 (1994) p. x.
[74] Warden.

interests, so long as immediate costs had the appearance of being controlled in order to sustain the drive towards managed care.

III. 7. COMPETITION. CONTAGION

Marketplace competition assumes that people are both rational and act only in self-interest. That competitive markets and 'evolution' of the market will eliminate errors by marketplace competition is assumed, even though little evidence supports these theoretical ideas while abundant evidence and everyday observations demonstrate the opposite. Yet, 'classical' economic theory of perfect rationality and self-interest does not account for departures from classical theory under uncertainty and under condition of imperfect knowledge, i.e. limited by bounded rationality and non-selfish behavior. The advocacy of medicine-on-the-cheap goes against a long history of economic theory. In 1622, Gerard Malynes said in *Lex Mercatoria*, "Strive not to undersell others to the hurt of the Commonwealth, under colour to increase trade: for trade doth not increase when commodities are good cheap, because the cheapness proceedeth of the small request and scarcity of money, which maketh things cheap: so that the contrary augmenteth trade, when there is plenty of money, and commodities become dearer being in request." Examples of departures from 'perfect competition' are legion, yet many economists prefer to presume that the marketplace must behave as a competitive market in continuous equilibrium.[75]

Managed care was based on assumptions that marketplace forces and competition would both hold down costs and improve quality. "Buying" health care did not meet necessary conditions for fair application of market competition, because patients were at mercy of their employers who were insulated from actions of managed care plans. Purchasers of managed care plans were dissociated from consumers, i.e. patients; the interest of both buyer and seller was cost.[76] If

---

[75] Lawrence M. Ausubel. "The Failure of Competition in the Credit Card Market." *American Economic Review* 81 (1991) 50-81. in Richard H. Thaler. *Advances in Behavioral Finance*, New York: Russell Sage, 1993 pp. 527-582; Thomas Russell and Richard Thaler. "The Relevance of Quasi Rationality in Competitive Markets." *American Economic Review* 75 (1985) 1071-1082; Herbert A. Simon. "Rational Decision Making in Business Organizations." *American Economic Review* 69 (1979) 493-513; Gerard Malynes. *Lex Mercatoria*, cited in John Maynard Keynes. *The General Theory of Employment, Interest, and Money*. Reprint. Amherst, NY: Prometheus, 1997, p. 344.

[76] A.S. Relman. "Shattuck Lecture—The Health Care Industry: Where is it Taking Us?" *New England Journal of Medicine* 325 (1991) 854-859; Susan Brink and Nancy Shute. "Managed care is pushing aside the private-practice doctors typified by TV's Marcus Welby or Dr.

the market approach to medical care was to succeed, competition must be present. Most health care delivery departs substantially from such competition, sometimes as a result of deliberate public or private policy. Perfect competition occurs when the individual seller or a buyer is so small relative to the total market that actions of a seller or a buyer do not affect market price. The most pressure came from large buyers of health care who exerted economic power against providers of health care, which was not the same as competition.[77]

Those people not in managed care plans also paid a price of managed care due to decreased availability of their doctors, and reduction in personnel and services in hospitals and other providers. Even nonprofit managed care companies, the alleged crusaders for patient-centered health care, were attacked for skimping on care to stay competitive.[78] Ruskin says, "Anarchy and competition, eternally, and in all things, [are] the laws of death."[79]

Claims made to justify managed care amounted to magical thinking, which has many parallels with movements in today's academic institutions. Magical thinking takes resemblance and/or co-occurrence as indicating a link or causal relationship between two objects or actions or events, such as fee-for-service solely the cause of rising costs. Anthropologists recognize that magical thinking does not distinguish primitive societies from technologically advanced ones, but is a feature of intellectual activity observed in all societies.[80] By forming part of a mass movement, a man descends several rungs on the ladder of civilization. Isolated, he may be a cultivated individual; in a mass, he is a creature acting by instinct. He possesses the spontaneity, the ferocity, and also the enthusiasm, and rarely heroism, of primitive beings whom he resembles by being impressed by words and images, which would be without action on isolated individuals composing the mass, and induced to commit acts contrary to his most obvious interests.[81]

Enthusiasm for managed care ran unchecked in the madness of a crowd, or mass behavior of the "collective subconscious of the primal horde" in which the

Kildare. What's replacing them isn't making anyone smile." *U.S. News and World Report* Oct 13, 1997.

[77] Erich H. Loewy. "Guidelines, Managed Care, and Ethics." *Archives of Internal Medicine* 156 (1996) 2038-2040.

[78] Victor R. Fuchs. "The 'Competition Revolution' in Health Care." *Health Affairs* 7 Summer (1988) 5-24.

[79] John Ruskin. *Ruskin Today.* from *Modern Painters V*, part Viii, chap. 1 (1860) London: Penguin, 1964, p. 275.

[80] James E. Alcock. "The Propensity to Believe." in *The Flight From Science and Reason.* Paul R. Gross, Norman Levitt, & Martin W. Lewis, editors. *Annals of New York Academy of Science.* vol. 775. (1996) p. 69.

[81] Le Bon. pp. 12-13.

will of an individual was too weak to venture upon any independent action.[82] In manias of banking and finance that parallel those of managed care, spread of euphoria from one market to another is readily understood—the bandwagon is under way: all climb aboard.[83]

The marketplace, production-line model of medical care that was expected to produce great savings as well as improve care was tested and failed, which led to a market-oriented health care system "spinning out of control." Nevertheless, a managed care spokesperson said that managed care is "not just a business—it's a movement."[84]

III. 8. FROM MADNESS TO MIRACLE TO MYTH

Self-contempt of individuals in mass movements produces the most unjust and criminal passions: he conceives a mortal hatred against that truth which blames him and convinces him of his faults.[85] Such excesses, based on fallacious and failed "intellectual underpinnings" of the irrational mass movement of managed care, led to persistence in error, i.e. folly. To qualify as folly, the policy adopted must meet three criteria:

1. Perceived as counter-productive in its own time, not in hindsight. The failed concepts of managed care have been known to be false for three decades.

2. A feasible alternative action must have been available, such as fee-for-service practice.

3. The policy in question should be that of a group, not an individual, and persist beyond one political lifetime.[86] The advocacy of managed care spans seven American presidential administrations.

Folly is independent of era or locality; it is timeless and universal, although habits and beliefs of a particular time and place determine the form it takes. Impotence of reason has wide-ranging effects because folly affects everything in a society.[87]

---

[82] Sigmund Freud. *Group Psychology and the Analysis of the Ego*. 1921. p. 686.
[83] Kindleberger. p. 103.
[84] Brink and Shute. Oct 13, 1997.
[85] Hoffer. p. 89.
[86] Tuchman. p. 5.
[87] Tuchman. p. 6.

Managed care was characterized as a 'miracle' by members of the health care consulting industry on a logically structured argument based on false assumptions and failed promises. From a concept without proof to a miracle required a true believer. Thus, managed care assumed the form of a mythic structure such that an advocate of the managed care mass movement exclaimed, "And, surely, from the enormous savings that have been made through this revolution [managed care mass movement], we also will be able to find an incremental way to provide access to basic health care for all our people,"[88] towards a vague, splendid future.

By myth, I do not mean false or meaningless, but a society's beliefs upon which it acts. In this respect, myth is more powerful than argument, objective evidence, or any sort of perceived truth to become its own version of truth. Myths are authoritative and truth-defining. Belief in performance of pre-admission and prior-authorization rituals became mythic. Myths are neither true nor false; they are useful fictions which fulfill social functions. Accepted myths or belief structures can be altered or discarded by an alternative belief. It was better to hold beliefs about the managed care industry critically than uncritically, even if it caused ambiguity and risk. Managed care advocates were highly sensitive to inquiry and criticism that might abase the myth. Articles alleging to show a vast difference in outcomes and costs favoring managed care over regular fee-for-service practice became part of the myth of managed care. A myth retains its sanction as long as it fits societal needs. Once the myth is no longer considered useful, it is discarded, replaced by a new and more satisfactory myth or belief.

Our 'uniform experience' aligns against miracle; otherwise it would not be a miracle. A miracle is therefore the most improbable of all events: it is always more probable that witnesses were lying or mistaken than a miracle occurred.[89] Lies extolling managed care were told so often, so stridently, and so insistently they became part of modern mythology, such that a proponent of managed care exclaimed managed care was a "bold and successful experiment."[90] That the managed care myth was based on false assumptions no longer mattered until tested by experience. The most sustained belief in miracles is the miracle of healing; managed care was the opposite. Miracles excite fear and wonder among spectators—which is what the word miracle implies—and are taken as evidence of supernatural power, until discarded. Nevertheless, the myth persisted, as a

---

[88] Paul M. Ellwood, Jr., and George D. Lundberg. "Managed Care: A Work in Progress." *Journal of the American Medical Association* 276 (1996) 1083-1086.
[89] C.S. Lewis. *Miracles*. New York: Macmillan, 1947. pp. 101-102.
[90] Ellwood and Lundberg. (1996).

proponent of the mass movement said in 1996: "As we go forward" with the managed care myth.[91]

Effectiveness of the doctrine of a mass movement does not come from its meaning or rationality but from its claim of certitude: the one and only truth. A doctrine must *not* be understood, but believed in. We can be absolutely certain about things we do not understand: a doctrine that is understood is shorn of its strength: "Once we understand a thing, it is as if it had originated in us....those who are asked to renounce the self and sacrifice it cannot see eternal certitude in anything which originates in that self."[92]

---

[91] Ellwood and Lundberg. (1996).
[92] Hoffer. p. 76.

Chapter IV

FINANCES OF THE MANAGED CARE INDUSTRY

The business community claimed that it was handicapped by costs of providing medical insurance for workers and their families, however, employers did not actually bear the cost of health insurance, but regarded it as a "useful myth" for selling universal coverage to an unwilling and unsuspecting public. Health expenditures have no more relationship to business competitiveness than do expenditures for hotels, transportation, or food prices. Employer contributions to health insurance are part of a total compensation package that includes basic wage rates, overtime payments, and fringe benefits. As long as total compensation is consistent with productivity, competitiveness is not affected. Employers told employees that they were "giving" them health insurance, in fact, health insurance was no more a gift than wages. In addition, health insurance, like other fringe benefits, is exempt from federal and state income taxes, Social Security contributions, and other payroll taxes. Workers prefer tax-free compensation whenever possible.[1]

We read that big managed care health plans were cash-rich, immensely wealthy, overwhelmingly powerful, and couldn't fail. An examination of finances of managed care health plans disclosed a surprising story:

Prior to 1993, average earnings growth of managed care plans was about 15 percent annually, or higher. Pre-tax profits were about 4 to 5 percent with an enrollment growth of about 10 percent per year. In 1993, managed care premiums on average rose 8 to 10 percent, but the expected increase in health care costs of 8 to 10% did not occur and were only 4 to 5%. Profits were embarrassingly large, beating managed care plans' expectations by wide margins. In 1994, managed

---

[1] V.R. Fuchs. "The Clinton Plan: A Researcher Examines Reform." *Health Affairs* 13 Spring (1994) 102-114.

care plans halved their rate of premium increases in 4 to 5 percent, while cost deceleration continued at only 0 to 1 percent, which caused profits to soar even more. Average pre-tax profit increased from 4 to 5 percent in 1991 to almost 12 percent by mid-1994. At the same time, membership grew at a rate of 20 percent and as high as 100 percent in some plans. The rush was on!

The sudden and sharp deflation in health care costs in 1993-1994 was true for the entire health care industry—both managed care *and* fee-for-service—a time when overall inflation in the economy declined. Since managed care plans accounted for only 15 percent of all health care, managed care plans were not the sole reason for decelerating costs in the entire health care industry because they were too small to have that much effect.

Physicians temporarily changed their practices when health care reform rhetoric was at its height resulting in industry-wide slowdown in physician visits, pharmaceutical and medical device pricing, and, to some degree, hospital visits and pricing. Both managed care plans and traditional fee-for-service plans experienced a doubling of profits in 1993-1994. The favorable health care inflation trend reversed in 1995, resulting in an inflation trend of 4 to 5 percent. Increase in costs plateaued towards the end of 1995, but it did not go down to 0 to 1 percent of 1994, as had been expected. When new members were recruited, new members signed up at premiums lower than that of existing members, which lowered average annual premiums.

New members were profitable to managed care companies because they typically don't fully utilize the new health plan, usually only 75 to 80 percent of true costs in the first year, so that health care costs were less for new members. Full utilization does not occur until at least the second year because new members take time to get accustomed to the new plan and its doctors. By the second year, they more fully utilize the plan. In this case, new members represent a sizable part of the total, and subsidize true costs: expenses would be less than revenues for a time, and profits would not decline to their true levels. That is, maturing obligations must be paid with new money.

New members came into managed care plans in 1995 at premium rates lower than the existing membership, with premiums lower than in 1994. In late 1994 and in 1995, managed care plans drew down their financial reserves, which artificially lowered health care expenses and helped managed care plans show better earnings growth than they actually had. Since reserves had been depleted, reserves were not available to boost managed care plans' financial results. If premiums lag health care costs after a year of severe price-cutting by even a moderate amount, a managed care plan must double or ever quadruple its enrollment to maintain the same level of profit.

The "seasoning phenomenon" allowed managed care companies to show good earnings growth up to a point; if price competition becomes sufficiently severe, gradual reduction in premiums (and resulting rise in the 'medical loss ratio') cannot be hidden, and rate of earnings growth falls even with strong enrollment growth. Examples of this phenomenon were US Healthcare, Humana, Coventry, Physicians Corp. of America, and a number of others, including Kaiser *Permanente*. Depending on how much financial reserves a managed care company built into its medical claims payable, a managed care company could mask underlying trends by drawing on its medical claims payable to artificially lower health care costs on its income statement, and prop-up earnings for awhile which enabled many managed care companies to report some earning grow in 1995.

Managed care plans had a membership attrition of about 15 percent who were rated at higher premiums than premiums of new members who became the new existing membership paying lower premiums than old members. Premiums in areas with the appearance of many new managed care plans were cut by as much as 4 to 5 percent. The alleged ability of managed care industry to hold down cost increases was discredited by Kaiser *Permanente* demanding a 12 percent or more increase in its premiums from some of its customers in June 1998. When one large client balked, it settled for a 10.75% increase.[2]

Medicare managed care was an unknown. In Medicare, 9.8 percent of all beneficiaries (due to more chronic illnesses) account for 68.4 percent of all Medicare costs.[3] Medicare HMO start-up costs are sizable and must be offset by enrollment of Medicare patients of at least 10,000. Medicare members tend to be older and consume more health care resources, so that a managed care company must have a large minimum membership to offset higher utilization by those who are sick. Unlike commercial groups, Medicare marketing was one-to-one, often in the potential members' homes, which required multiple visits to obtain signed contracts. Starting Medicare managed care programs proved to be very expensive with substantial losses the first year or two.

To compete, managed care companies offered inducements at no extra premium, such as hearing aids, glasses, prescription drugs, etc., which was disastrous to more than one managed care company. Accepting a meant enrollees needed it, and consumed more additional medical services. A 'medical loss ratio' of 90 to 95 percent was common when a managed care company entered a new market. In 1995, Physicians Corp. of America had Medicare 'medical losses ratio'

[2] Carl T. Hall. "Huge Loss For Kaiser—Rates to Rise." *San Francisco Chronicle* 14 Feb 1996.
[3] Joel M. Karlin. "Managed care prompts a lesson in cooperation." *American Medical News* Oct. 21, 1996.

of 95 to 110-plus percent. Other managed care companies experienced Medicare start up losses as high as 120 percent. When a managed care company entered a new market, its premium rates were too low to generate profits or to implement sophisticated cost controls.[4] During 1996, many large managed care plans posted lower earnings than the year before.[5] Thus, the managed care industry itself showed signs of aging and had to be sustained by new money.

In managed care, providers supposedly "share risk" with the managed care plan, when in fact all risk was born by doctors, hospitals and other suppliers of medical services. Managed care companies were guaranteed their profit and expenses. In the case of bad luck, known in managed care as "adverse experience," "medical losses" or an excess of claims for the sick and injured, doctors and hospitals bore the added costs. Re-insurance by providers may or may not cover part of excess expenses.[6]

Most physicians did not recognize that division into was a road to serfdom. Managed care managers became literal "bounty hunters" who were allowed to carve out enormous profit margins for themselves. Government and business payers took no notice allowing managed care companies to keep up to 30 cents of premium dollars for administration, marketing and profit.[7] A few "gloated" over disorganization of physicians, and some contended that large fraction of revenues spent on marketing, administration and profits was what would be expected of any business.[8]

QualMed HMO in Northern California was 'sold' in 1992 for 45 times earnings, or three times a reasonable price, a tactic known on Wall Street as the 'jelly-roll,' a way to create an image of great potential future worth—betting on a long-shot.

Humana drew on a $1.5 billion line of credit from Chase Manhattan Bank to finance acquisitions. Rather than cash-rich, managed care companies financial status was based on an increasing long-term debt. In the 1996, Humana struggled with cost cutting, withdrew from unprofitable HMOs in Washington, and

[4] Kimberly A. Purvis. "Health Maintenance Organizations: Why Our Short-Term View on the HMOs Remains Negative." *Industry Viewpoint*. Donaldson, Lufkin & Jenrette. New York, NY Jan. 10, 1996.
[5] *APC Inv. Rel Corp Finance*. Dow Jones & Co., 10/21/96.
[6] "Background Paper for Capitation Hearing." California Legislature, Senate Committee on Judiciary. June 6, 1995.
[7] John K. Iglehart. "Health Policy Report: The Struggle Between Managed Care and Fee-for-Service Practice." *New England Journal of Medicine* 331 (1994) 63-67.
[8] Jerome P. Kassirer. "The Business of Managed Care." *San Francisco Chronicle* Aug 15, 1995.

Alabama, eliminated 700 jobs, and replaced top company officials, including the president and chief financial officer.[9]

Annual financial reports of managed care companies yield more surprising information, that the managed care industry was something other than financial powerhouses we had been led to believe. Evaluating the financial state of managed care entities can be made by comparison with other types of insurance[10]: the 'prudential rule' of insurance requires one cycle of claims in reserves of cash or equivalents. In health care insurance, the cycle between collection of premiums and payment of claims is about three months; thus, a managed care company must have thirteen weeks of premiums in cash reserves to be considered solvent.

PHP Healthcare Corporation, (Annual Report 1996) had been in business almost 25 years in the Washington, DC area. Average net income 1992 through 1996 was reported as a negative 0.15%. Cash reserves in 1995 amounted to two days of expenses, versus the thirteen weeks of premium revenues an insurance company must have to satisfy the 'prudential rule of solvency.' In 1996, PHP reported 12.3 weeks of cash reserves—a surprising "turn-around" when gross revenues decreased by 0.5 percent. PHP's increase in "cash and equivalents" came from the sale of $65.4 million of stock. Without sale of stock, the company would have had a negative "cash and equivalents," or no cash reserves. PHP's stock price dropped in two years from $28 to as low as $0.05 in 1999.

An example of volatility of the managed care industry occurred in the Fall of 1997 when the price of stock of Oxford Health Care managed care company dropped more than 62% on the day when Dow Jones Industrial average dropped 7%. Oxford's earnings and share price had quadrupled since 1994 on strength of robust membership growth and innovative marketing that had been the envy of the managed care industry. Three months earlier, Oxford shares achieved a 52-week high of $89. The managed care industry was struggling with higher medical costs, the challenge of large mergers, and public concerns over whether managed care companies were denying care to patients to hold down costs. Oxford blamed its woes on problems linked to a new computer system that led it to overestimate revenue and membership enrollment, and underestimate costs of medical care, a familiar excuse given by many types of business after a decline in corporate performance to blame their own failures and folly on computer systems. In August 1997, insiders of Oxford Health Corporation sold millions of dollars of stock. Complaints of long delays in reimbursement were growing; Oxford booked

[9] Milt Freudenheim. "Humana Buys Health Plan In Cincinnati." *New York Times* June 6, 1997.
[10] John L. Akula. "Insolvency Risk in Health Carriers: Innovation, Competition, and Public Protection." *Health Affairs* 6 Jan/Feb (1997) 9-32.

revenues for members they didn't have.[11] In February 1998, Oxford Health obtained "badly needed capital" from two buy-out firms of $300 million in equity financing and $300 million in additional debt in exchange for the buy-out firms owning 15 to 20 percent of Oxford Health Plan, acquiring more debt in an effort to survive its falling performance and failed promise.[12]

In 1996, PacifiCare Health Systems announced plans to acquire FHP for "$2.1 billion in cash and stock." PacifiCare executives claimed merger would result in economies of scale, significant savings on overhead and better services to managed care plan members. Critics said that mergers came at the expense of patients "already victimized" by HMO cost cutting.[13] According to *PacifiCare Health Systems Annual Report 1995*, its average net income 1986 through 1995 was 2.1 percent; average number of weeks of cash reserves averaged 10.7 weeks which is below the thirteen weeks considered 'prudent' for a health insurance company. In 1995, PacifiCare listed assets of $1.39 billion of which $296 million (21.4%) was listed as "Goodwill," another device that creates a false value; in 1996, its long term debt of $1.13 billion and goodwill of $2.53 billion. By the end of 1997, *PacifiCare's* long term debt had grown from $3.3 million in 1987 to $1.1 billion, and at the same time reported a loss of $21 million—another example of losing money while growing in enrollees and revenues: a time that is usually the most profitable for managed care plans. Cash and equivalents were reported to be 8.9 weeks of annual premiums, well below the thirteen weeks required for solvency. One half of *PacifiCare's* assets were listed as "goodwill." *PacifiCare* drew $1.1 billion on a $1.5 billion line of credit with a balloon payment due in the year 2001: a consistent story in the managed care industry, not florid with cash so much as laden with debt.

Despite the record, chief executive officers of managed care companies on the average were paid 62 percent more than chief executive officers of comparable sized corporations. Mergers and take-overs generated fortunes for executives in the managed care industry. Managed care companies were criticized for too much going to administration and profit, and too little to provide patient care.[14]

The stage was set for a financial crisis in the managed care industry. In such cases, we may look at other areas of finance to see what happens in such circumstances.[15] The boom of a new enterprise is fed by bank credit which is

[11] Ron Winslow. "Oxford to Post First Quarterly Loss Ever." *Wall Street Journal* 10-28-97.
[12] *San Francisco Chronicle* 2-13-98.
[13] Carl T. Hall. "$2.1 Billion Deal Creates Huge HMO." *San Francisco Chronicle.* Aug 6, 1996.
[14] Thomas Bodenheimer. "The HMO Backlash—Righteous or Reactionary?" *New England Journal of Medicine* 335 (1996) 1601-1604.
[15] Charles P. Kindleberger. *Manias, Panics, and Crashes: A History of Financial Crises.* Third Edition. New York, Chichester, Brisbane, Toronto, Singapore: John Wiley, 1996. p. 11.

notoriously unstable. Demand exceeds capacity to supply, and gives rise to profit opportunities, such that "euphoria" of speculation further increasing prices. Euphoria leads to over-estimation of profits, attracting investors who normally would avoid such ventures because speculation leads away from normal, rational behavior to 'manias' or 'bubbles'—an upward price movement over an extended range that implodes, and extended negative bubble results in a crash.[16]

At late stage, speculation tends to detach itself from real value and turns to delusions of value; more people seek to become rich without understanding risks: "Not surprisingly, swindlers and catchpenny schemes flourish." At top of a speculative market, hesitation occurs as new recruits to speculation balance insiders who withdraw. A period of financial distress follows where a company must face the possibility that it will not be able to meet its liabilities, which often leads to a rush to recover liquidity—money—from speculation leaving speculative borrowers unable to pay their loans. Speculators come to realize that the market cannot go higher, and a race out of investment into cash turns into a stampede. The signal that precipitates a crisis may be failure of a bank or firm stretched too far, revelation of a "swindle or defalcation" by someone who sought to escape by dishonest means, or fall in price of the object of speculation as it is seen to be overpriced, then results in 'revulsion' from mania as panic feeds on itself.[17] Kindleberger sardonically observes, "These incurable optimists, who know they are going to win the first time, but lose, frequently try again, often doubling their bets and enlarging their risks by operations of dubious morality or evident illegality."[18] In 1997, stockholdings by the managed care industry increased over 100 percent as managed care companies attempted to support failing profits with money taken away from providing care: a risky course in the face of an already long bull market and market volatility.[19]

Conversion to managed care had potential to pressure hospitals to the point they could not fund debt service on their capital loans, or provide many community services, such as care for the uninsured,[20] which contrasted with realities of a market society which requires that corporate business managers have no responsibility except to maximize profits to shareholders: shareholders can sue corporate executives who sacrifice profits for ethics.[21]

---

[16] Kindleberger. p. 13.
[17] Kindleberger. p. 15.
[18] Kindleberger. p. 73.
[19] Chris Rauber. "HMO study finds $780 million loss." *Modern Healthcare*. Sept. 7, 1998. pp. 24, 30.
[20] Kassirer.
[21] David U. Himmelstein and Steffie Woolhandler. "Bound to Gag." *Archives of Internal Medicine* 157 (1997) 2033.

Health Net, whose parent company was Health Systems International [HSI], was one of the companies used to illustrate massive financial power of the managed care industry. Health Net was formed in 1979 by Blue Cross of Southern California; merger of QualMed and Health Net made CEO Roger Greaves and others wealthy overnight by transforming non-profit Health Net into a for-profit company.[22] Premium money flowed in so fast that at one time it had $475 million to invest with $500,000 coming in each day.[23]

In 1995 with $500 million in assets, Health Net appeared awesome, however $275 million was listed as 'goodwill.' In addition, HSI had $175 million in long term debt and applied for a $400 million line of credit. HSI's stock price at the time ranged from $30 to $35, however its book value was only $0.86. HSI is no newcomer, yet its Standard and Poor rating in July 1995 was NR: "Not Rated," a designation reserved for new stock listings or those that are nearly insolvent. *Health Systems International* [Health Net], *Annual Report 1995* lists premium revenue of $2,692 million, with a net income of $89.6 million, or income of 3.3 percent. It purchased M.D. Enterprises of Connecticut, the third largest HMO in the state, for "approximately $100 million in cash" which made Health Net sound cash rich. However, *Report* states that the company borrowed $100 million from a $400 million line of credit to fund the MDEC acquisition, i.e. the alleged "cash" purchase was made with borrowed money.[24] In 1996, Health Systems International merged with Foundation Health Corporation. By 1997, the combined debt of HSI and FHP grew in five years 1992 to 1996 from $56 million to $754.2 million!

In 1997, the new company, called 'Foundation Health Systems,' reported premium income of $5.83 billion and a loss of $89.3 million during a time of considerable growth in enrollees, the time when profits are expected to be highest. Merger costs were reported as $70.4 million so that merger costs did not account for its loss for the year. The scapegoat of computer related expenses was duly employed. Of total assets of $4 billion, one fourth was noted as 'goodwill.' Cash and equivalents were 9.9 weeks, below the 13 weeks required for solvency. It was now operating under a revolving line of credit of $1.5 billion from which it had borrowed $1.3 billion. Although it grew with new enrollees, Foundation Health Systems, too, lost money while growing during the years that ordinarily produce the greatest profits. By the end of 1998, FHC's *10-K Annual Report* shows that gross revenues for the year were $8,896 million; its long term debt increased to

[22] Erik Larson. "The Soul of an HMO." *Time* Jan. 22, 1996, pp. 45-52.
[23] George Anders. *Health Against Wealth: HMOs and the Breakdown of Medical Trust.* Boston and New York: Houghton Mifflin, 1996, p. 63.
[24] *Form 10-K Annual Report: Year Ending Dec 31, 1996: Health Systems International, Inc.* p. 42.

$1,530 million; and its income a negative $165 million. FHC's cash and equivalent reserves had dropped to $78 million or 3.2 days of revenues as opposed to 13 weeks required for solvency.

The wealth of the managed care industry is, therefore, in paper, and depends on anticipated massive, future earnings for solvency, which appear unlikely to be realized. Many managed care executives took their rewards in stock certificates that were redeemable only if the stock reached targeted and usually very high prices. Although often considered one of the 'big players,' Health Systems/Foundation appears in the same condition as other managed care companies: its riches in paper, and burdened with debt, including Kaiser *Permanente*. After losing $447 million in 1997, Kaiser *Permanente* lost $434 million in 1998 reducing its reserves to a few weeks, while only a few HMOs reported small profits.[25]

The mass movement into managed care gained momentum and advanced on these financial misconceptions:

- Business representative wrongly claimed the nations businesses were hampered in international competition by the costs of medical care.
- Managed care did not lower costs of health care insurance.
- Managed care plans were "highly leveraged," i.e., acquired enormous long-term debt.
- An unusually strong economy and stock market sustained financial backing for the managed care industry.
- During growth in enrollees, managed care plans lost money.

Corporatization of health care was aptly described as a "market-driven mess."[26] The bubble of the managed care industry grew ever larger.

---

[25] R.D. Smith. *Managed Care: Anatomy of a Mass Medical Movement.* Bristol, IN: Wyndham Hall Press, 2000, pp. 272-273.
[26] Kassirer.

Chapter V

CAUTIONS

V. 1. RESISTANCE

In the past, criticism of Kaiser *Permanente* and the managed care industry became a sanction. As the rush towards managed care gained momentum, resistance to its endorsement began to be heard. Liberal politicians were as skeptical of a system dominated by managed care as were some conservative fee-for-service doctors fearing that it would neglect the poor in order to maximize profits at expense of medical care.[1] Patients with long standing relationships with their doctors had to choose new doctors under managed care plans; for doctors, shifts of long-time patients affected his or her ability to earn a livelihood.[2]

Enthusiasm for cost-cutting potential of managed care reflected aggressive industry public relations more than actual results. Most studies claiming to show a significant managed-care advantage failed to account adequately for key factors affecting health-insurance costs. Whatever savings were possible from managed care was a one-time event. In order to prevent over-use of medical services by patients, care was 'managed' by thousands of administrators, enforcing rules and regulations on patients and providers. Costs of Federal Employees Health Benefits Plan (FEHBP) in managed care rose 25 percent greater than premiums in fee-for-service during the 1980s. Aggressive efforts toward cost control led to complaints of rationing.[3]

---

[1] John K. Iglehart. "Health Policy Report: The Struggle Between Managed Care and Fee-for-Service Practice." *New England Journal of Medicine* 331 (1994) 63-67.

[2] "Background Paper for Capitation Hearing." California Legislature. Senate Committee on Judiciary. Senator Charles M. Calderon, Chairman. June 6, 1995.

[3] John Merline. "Pay or Pay: Managed care will not save Medicare, but a dose of reality might." *National Review* May 29, 1995, pp. 45-48.

Practices of the managed care industry appeared at odds with ideals of ethical medical practice, challenged as to whether managed care companies adhered to Medical Code of Ethics or acted in public interest, citing patients' rights to make their own choice of physicians, physicians' rights to direct their own patients to appropriate specialists, preservation of unobstructed physician-patient communications, and maintenance of a medical delivery system capable of meeting medical needs of a community. Managed care was able to undermine care by exclusion of physicians, restriction of free trade, and suppression of free speech, which was erroneously called "reform."[4]

"Reform" strategy displaced people into HMOs, restricted choice of physicians and hospitals, and used gatekeepers to curb referrals to specialists and technologically advanced diagnosis and treatment. Missing was elimination of the 'withhold,' a pervasive managed care practice of punishing doctors for providing care they believed their patients needed. Almost all large, for-profit managed care companies withheld between 10 percent and 25 percent of doctors' compensation until year's end and returned it only if HMOs' targets for costs were reached by limiting patients' tests, referrals to specialists, and hospitalizations. Targets were so stringent that HMOs almost always keep part, or all, of the withhold—a practice that led to a surge in "hallway consultations" in order to avoid referring patients to specialists. By destroying reciprocal rights of the physician-patient relationship, integral to ethical medical care, the managed care industry transformed medical care into a commodity-market ethic. The same was true for physicians' relations with one another. Honesty and trust on both sides of the physician-patient relationship remained extremely important,[5] and was seriously jeopardized by managed care.

"Utilization review" added to burdens of obtaining timely care in which delays occurred while doctors obtained authorizations from a review company to proceed with diagnostic and treatment plans which were reviewed by a clerk or a nurse stationed at a computer. Three hundred fifty utilization review companies claiming to slash health care costs sold their services to managed care companies amounting to a $7 billion industry advocating "cookbook medicine." Even when doctors' recommendations were ultimately approved, it took several weeks longer to diagnose and begin treating a managed care patient than a patient under fee-for-service insurance because of successive delays in getting each step approved.

[4] Ronald A. Zumbrun. "Managed care vs. the medical code of ethics." *The Daily Recorder*. Sacramento, CA, March 13, 1995.
[5] Victor R. Fuchs. "Managed Care and Merger Mania." *Journal of the American Medical Association* 277 (1997) 920-921.

Further objections arose against waste, duplication, and abuse in management of managed care.

During 1980s, a marked rise occurred in number of families in which both husband and wife were employed: that each was eligible for employment-related health benefits had important implications. In the San Francisco Bay Area, during decades of growth and sanction of Kaiser *Permanente*, many families had double coverage: going to a Kaiser *Permanente* facility for routine medical matters, and consulting a private fee-for-service doctor when in need of care which distorted claims of cost-control by promoters of managed care. Further, competition has not been more effective in keeping costs down than any other approach.[6] That both patient and physician have free choice in a voluntary relationship was impossible because many patients cannot make free choices since they must consider cost of care, implications of loss of health insurance, and rules of managed care networks that limit their options.[7] When business groups formed to deal with managed care companies, they discovered a wide disparity in premiums charged by managed care plans for similar businesses, and concluded that managed care plans charged businesses whatever they could-get-away-with.[8] Managed care plans combined insurance function with delivery function, a dangerous mix when managed care markets were saturated with costs still rising: financial ruin could be averted only by reducing quality and breadth of services "endangering the health of individuals, families, or whole communities."[9]

V. 2. ROLE OF THE MANAGED CARE INSURANCE INDUSTRY

Group selection, risk selection, risk management, cappers, steerers, shadow pricing were standard practices of the managed care industry, such as 'blue lining' to exclude those in an undesirable demographic category, and 'cherry picking' selecting the young and healthy.

Agencies that were expected to assume and plan for risk in medical insurance became adept at *avoiding* risk. Claims for expensive procedures may or may not

---

[6] A.S. Relman. "Assessment and Accountability: The Third Revolution in Medical Care." *New England Journal of Medicine* 319 (1988) 1220-1222.

[7] Robert O'Brien. "The Doctor-Patient Relationship." in *Beyond the Crisis: Preserving the Capacity for Excellence in Health Care and Medical Science* Henry M. Greenberg and Susan U. Raymond, editors. *Annals of the New York Academy of Sciences* 729, 1994. p. 23.

[8] Brian O'Reilly. "Taking on the HMOs." *Fortune* Feb 16, 1998, pp. 96-104.

[9] John H. McArthur and Francis D. Moore. "The Two Cultures and the Health Care Revolution: Commerce and Professionalism." *Journal of the American Medical Association* 277 (1997) 985-989.

be denied on the basis of protection of profits. Certain methods of rejecting claims for treatment appeared to be pervasive, such as excluding procedures as experimental, rejecting a claim whole or in part for procedural or technical reasons, making the claims process and its rules overly complex, drawing out the process in order to gain investment income on premiums held for as long as possible, and by inducing patients and physicians to give up. Delays in payment were important for insurance companies, because they gained high returns from investing premiums collected, a practice known as "working the float." Such tactics forced doctors and hospitals to hire additional personnel to fight claim-delays and harassment.

Selection by requiring attendance at sign-up sessions skimmed those who could get to the sign-up sites, which may be upstairs in a building with no elevator.[10] Clever underwriting to reduce risk by excluding pre-existing conditions for a year or more is now limited by state law, nevertheless, managed care plans asked 43 percent of Medicare applicants about their health status which was illegal, with the net effect that healthy elderly patients migrated into managed care plans leaving sicker patients in traditional Medicare driving up its costs. The shift from physicians' offices to institution-based care raised objections to the transparent financial incentives of providing too little care.[11]

Open enrollment was the single provision of the 1973 HMO Act that was "more firmly and vociferously" opposed by the managed care industry, as well as community rating which they feared might result in adverse selection over time and lead to financial disaster.[12] "Gag clauses" nakedly revealed who made decisions in managed care, contradicting their rhetoric of accountability.[13] Many suspected that 'managed care' meant 'managed billing' that raised costs as it lowered payments for medical services. Added costs and lost revenues associated with claim delays forced hospitals to increase charges to cover deficits.

Managed care companies became adept at underwriting to avoid covering high-risk populations altogether, called 'risk rating' or 'experience rating,' such as 'direct' risk rating, by avoiding coverage for pre-existing conditions, denying coverage for groups, or even whole occupations or industries. 'Indirect' risk rating was pervasive by extended waiting periods, writing new policies each year so that

[10] Philip R. Alper. "Medical Practice in the Competitive Market." *New England Journal of Medicine* 316 (1987) 337-339.

[11] Uwe E. Reinhardt. "Health System Change: Skirmish or Revolution?" *Health Affairs.* 15 Winter (1996) 114-115.

[12] Lawrence D. Brown. *Politics and Health Care Organization: HMOs as Federal Policy.* Washington, DC: The Brookings Institution, 1983. p. 304.

[13] David U. Himmelstein and Steffie Woolhandler. "Bound to Gag." *Archives of Internal Medicine* 157 (1997) 2033.

waiting periods started all over again ("policy churning"), raising deductibles, increasing co-payments, limiting amounts paid for procedures ("payment caps"), selectively designed benefits packages (e.g. limiting mental health coverage), and selective marketing to attract lower-risk prospects. Since about 75 percent of health care costs are associated with 10 percent of people who have the highest costs, an economist noted that for an insurer to design its plan to encourage bad risks to "enroll elsewhere" could be extremely advantageous.[14] Marketing strategies were designed to attract good risks and to avoid patients who would cost the plan money. Managed care advertisements typically displayed smiling elderly people fishing, traveling, and happy, healthy babies—not patients with congestive heart failure, cancer, or cerebral palsy on the grounds of their clinical excellence in treating them.[15]

Most people underestimated the magnitude of conflict between a physician functioning under traditional medical ethics and the same physician functioning under a managed care system because of irreducible conflict between 'cost-driven' opposed to 'care-driven' health care.[16] Delays in care, postponement of consultation or hospitalization, impersonality, loss of dignity, and magnification of suffering influenced quality of care, degree of satisfaction, and functional capacity of the ill were not resolvable under managed care.[17] A trade-off between competing goals of cost reduction, access, and satisfaction became unavoidable.[18] Many patients resisted changing doctors, preferred small offices to institution-based care, and objected to transparent financial incentives for providing too little care.[19] Further, the physician-patient relationship itself has therapeutic value.[20]

Managed care companies made large profits in areas where payments to Medicare managed care companies were high. Some plans paid physicians and other providers reasonably well for a time, which was a "teaser," an inducement, that lasted only until of doctor's Medicare patients had enrolled in the managed

[14] A.C. Enthoven. "Effective Management of Competition in the FEHBP." *Health Affairs* 8 Fall (1989) 33-50.

[15] Lynn Etheredge, Stanley B. Jones, and Lawrence Lewin. "What Is Driving Health System Change?" *Health Affairs* 15 Winter (1996) 93-104.

[16] E.D. Pelegrino. "Managed care and managed competition: some ethical reflections." *Calyx* 4 (1994) 1-5.

[17] Fred Rosner. "Managed Care: Ethical Issues." Letter. *Journal of the American Medical Association* 274 (1995) 609-610.

[18] John M. Eisenberg. "Economics." *Journal of the American Medical Association* 273 (1995) 1670-1671.

[19] Steffie Woolhandler and David Himmelstein. "Extreme Risk—The New Corporate Proposition for Physicians." *New England Journal of Medicine* 333 (1995) 1706-1708.

[20] Kathy S. Doner. "Managed Care: Ethical Issues." Letter. *Journal of the American Medical Association* 274 (1995) 609.

care HMO.[21] In areas where managed care plans were just taking hold, physicians were offered contracts that contained a clause that the managed care company could change reimbursements to doctors without their consent, fees were cut shortly after physicians signed on.[22] Some managed care plans were notoriously unreliable when verifying member eligibility or other costs. Inflationary causes in health care occurred with multiple competing insurance plans, each with it own overhead costs of marketing and administration.

Managed care was supposed to increase efficiency in medical care, and reduce costs, yet three of the biggest HMOs were the slowest to pay—as long as 94 days behind in payments to physicians and hospitals. Coincidentally or not, payment delays swelled the bottom lines of managed care companies. In 1995, managed care companies held on to unpaid claims for average of 89.5 days. Delays tended to be longer in areas with the most people in managed care plans. Large HMOs profited as much as $400,000 a day while collecting interest by holding on to funds of unpaid claims. In 2001, Pacificare was fined $250,000 and Heritage Provider Network $50,000 for late payments to providers. Health Net was fined $100,000 plus interest for late payments to providers for delays of up to one year, bills that are required to be paid within 45 days.[23]

Nevertheless, most proposals for national health insurance placed trillion-dollar health care financing in hands of the industry that proved its expertise at selecting risks, limiting coverage, and denying or delaying payments. The insurance industry was well aware that health insurance was not necessary in national health policy. The insurance industry poured billions into buying out delivery systems in order to have a major share of the market or a monopoly: doctors and hospitals felt they had to sell out or be excluded. Thus, insurance companies, not physicians, payers or employers, controlled the delivery of medical services: a central flaw of managed care and managed competition—its design undermined its purpose.[24]

Managed care plans used the phrase "medically necessary and appropriate care" which meant a doctor might recommend treatment and the managed care plan would not authorize it.[25] 'Medical necessity' to the managed care industry

[21] Ken Terry. "Don't miss out on Medicare managed care." *Medical Economics* April 7 (1997) 59-82.
[22] Mark Crane. "How low can fees go?" *Medical Economics* April 7 (1997) 26-47.
[23] Milt Freudenheim. "Dragging Out HMO Payments." *New York Times* April 17, 1997; Victoria Colliver. "Health Net Fined for Late Payments." *San Francisco Chronicle* 26 Sep 2001.
[24] Donald W. Light. "Life, Death, and the Insurance Companies." *New England Journal of Medicine* 330 (1994) 498-499.
[25] Susan Brink and Nancy Shute. "Managed care is pushing aside the private-practice doctors typified by TV's Marcus Welby or Dr. Kildare. What's replacing them isn't making anyone smile." *U.S. News and World Report* Oct 13, 1997.

meant whatever-they-could-get-away-with in delays and denial of care by abrogating public trust; and in the process, the managed care industry gained extraordinary force and momentum. Medical ethical standards that evolved over two millennia never envisioned a market-driven health care system with incentives to under-treat patients.[26] One can hardly consider the mass movement of managed care without being appalled by ethics and tactics of the managed care insurance industry. In irrational mass movements, malfeasance eventually comes to light and "raises revulsion, and perhaps discredit."[27]

A mass movement, such as managed care, is consolidated by practical men-of-action (the CEOs of the managed care companies and others) who save the movement from self-destructiveness and recklessness of zealots. Practical men and women-of-action are not thinkers, since they possess little capacity of foresight which might lead to doubt and inactivity, who are especially recruited from ranks of those "morbidly nervous, excitable, half-deranged persons who are bordering on madness." Their convictions are so strong that all reasoning is lost on them. Contempt and persecution do not affect them but excite them more. Men-of-action have no thought beyond realizing the accepted belief, legislators applying it, and men of letters solely preoccupied with its expression.[28]

The appearance of practical men and women-of-action marks the end of the dynamic phase of a mass movement when protest and desire for drastic change were dominant: the battle with the established order is over. The man-of-action becomes intent on possessing the new world, not renovating it, and in perpetuating his power won. The vigor of the mass movement is transferred to the movement's institutions: managed care companies. No longer can the mass movement rely on transient enthusiasm or persuasion, but it depends on drill and coercion on the assumption that all men are cowards, such that the movement maintains a steady flow of propaganda using old fear-engendering formulas and slogans, which were emphasized in the managed care mass movement by financial coercion. Earlier zealots and men-of-words are canonized in order to present the new order as the "glorious consummation of the hopes and struggles of the early days," with such claims in the managed care mass movement that "we have achieved a great deal," and that the mass movement of managed care was "a bold and successful experiment."[29]

[26] J.P. Kassirer. "Preserving Our Noble Heritage." *Western Journal of Medicine.* 164 (1996) 535-536.
[27] Charles P. Kindleberger. *Manias, Panics, and Crashes: A History of Financial Crises.* Third Edition. New York, Chichester, Brisbane, Toronto, Singapore: John Wiley, 1996, p. 82.
[28] Gustave Le Bon. *The Crowd: A Study of the Popular Mind.* (1895) Dunwoody, GA: Norman S. Berg, 2nd ed. 1984. pp. 113-115, 146.
[29] Paul M. Ellwood, Jr., and George D. Lundberg. "Managed Care: A Work in Progress." *Journal of the American Medical Association* 276 (1996) 1083-1086.

In 1999, Aetna US Healthcare coerced physicians into participating in all of their plans including HMOs in an all-or-nothing clause or dropped from all Aetna US Healthcare participation which would permit managed care plans to dictate all aspects of patient care and drive towards HMOs. A desire for the establishment of stability preoccupies a mass movement, so that the movement is no longer a refuge for self-realization or ambition: reconciliation with the present, rather than to posterity.[30] Thus, the militancy and control of the managed care companies and their case managers must have the threat of coercion, or the movement begins to fail.

V. 3. REGULATORY AGENCIES

For a mass movement such as managed care to gain momentum, regulatory agencies and government protective oversight mechanisms must be slack, and often complicit, in spread of the mass movement. The California Department of Corporations assumed regulatory responsibility for the managed care industry in 1975, by default when the Legislature enacted the Knox-Keene Act to license and regulate prepaid health plans which was then made up of Kaiser *Permanente* and a few smaller nonprofit plans with a total of 2.8 million members. Because the managed care industry feared legal and financial ramifications of being treated as insurance companies, it lobbied successfully against being regulated by the Department of Insurance, which would be the logical agency for managed care industry's regulation and oversight. Thus, regulation of the managed care industry fell to an agency that specialized in issuing business licenses and regulating investment firms.

In the 20 years it held jurisdiction over the managed care industry, the Department of Corporations fined a managed care company for violating patient care standards only once—a $500,000 fine imposed on TakeCare HMO in 1994. Beyond that single case, none of the state's ten biggest managed care companies had been cited by the Department of Corporations for a violation relating to patient care since at least 1985 when department records began. The Department of Corporations failed to exercise its responsibility that it inspect each HMO at least once every five years for compliance with state health and safety standards. Three of the state's biggest HMOs had never been audited. The Department of Corporations assisted the managed care industry in "throwing a curtain over

---

[30] Milt Freudenheim. "Insurers Moving to Limit Doctor's Contract Choices." *New York Times*. Feb. 8, 1999; Eric Hoffer. *The True Believer*. New York: Harper & Row, pp. 195,. 134-138.

problems and deficiencies that by law it must publicly disclose." The department disposed of as many as 90% of complaints about managed care by directing consumers back to HMOs' own grievance systems which were not required to have specific guidelines on how complaints were handled. The result, critics said, was the "appearance of HMO regulation—but not the reality." A former department investigator said that the "facade of being regulated" served a great benefit to the managed care industry, but in reality there was no regulation. Even when the department attempted to investigate, it was sometimes stonewalled by the managed care industry.

Sanctions against the managed care industry were not publicly disclosed, and a provision to eliminate secrecy of the findings of investigations was killed by the managed care lobby.[31] Most state regulators of the managed care industry considered their role was to promote managed care companies so as to "rein in" hospital and physician costs.[32] As one managed care plan surveyor confessed, "Our primary business is to sell the Kaisers and Aetnas and Cignas of the world. We don't want anything in print that would get them irritated."[33] Finally, in 2000, the California Department of Corporations fined Kaiser *Permanente* $1,000,000 for delay in urgent medical treatment due to "systemic health care delivery problems" and it was faulted for "failing to ensure that care be accessible to enrollees; failing to provide basic health care services including preventive and emergency care; and failing to have medical records readily available."[34]

So pervasive was the mass movement of managed care that universities and medical schools were caught-up in the mania of managed care; agents that should look critically at the managed care industry acted as opportunists in developing curricula promoting managed care that produced income for universities. The rush towards the mass movement of managed care and slack regulation by agencies and academic institutions that were charged with the responsibility to oversee and regulate served to promote and cover-up deficiencies of the mass movement of managed care.

In the regulatory activities, we see in action the fallacy of *The Official Malefactor's Screen*: "attack us—you attack the government."

---

[31] David R. Olmos and Michael A. Hiltzik. "State Oversight of HMOs Is Weak, Critics Charge." *Los Angeles Times* August 28, 1995.
[32] George Anders. *Health Against Wealth: HMOs and the Breakdown of Medical Trust.* Boston and New York: Houghton Mifflin, 1996, p. 230.
[33] Anders. p. 258.
[34] Julie Marquis. "Kaiser is fined $1million." *Contra Costa Times.* 16 May 2000.

V. 4. MASS MOVEMENT FEEDS ON ITSELF

When a mass movement attains enough momentum and public acceptance, it sustains itself with little further impetus. Critical faculties are no longer called upon, people surrender to the collective will of the mass, nothing stands in its way: the train has left the station, all are on board. Those with information and a duty to bring understanding became part of the movement. One medical journal editor claimed that all insurance subsidized by the government or business should be converted as rapidly as possible to managed care, and contract with "not-for-profit group-model HMOs that are managed jointly by physicians and members,"[35] affirming that managed care was truly the future of medical practice.

In 1996, others exclaimed that the most important new pressure on providers would be the "rapid movement of Medicare enrollees into managed care,"[36] asserting that the battle was over and managed care proponents succeeded, that it was hopeless to resist. The bubble grew without restraint by ignoring failed concepts and overt misrepresentation of the management of managed care; a 'bubble' appears as the result of "herd behavior, positive feedback or bandwagon effects—credulous suckers…" flocked to the mass movement of managed care.

The individual in a mass undergoes a profound mental change: emotions are extraordinarily intensified, while intellectual ability becomes markedly reduced in approximation to other individuals of the group, the result of removal of inhibitions of instincts peculiar to each individual, and by resigning expressions of his own.[37] Masses lose sight of realities; they overestimate their strength, are greedy for a share in anticipated distribution of power, and, ruled as they are by prejudice, project their own anti-social tendencies onto fictitious adversaries, i.e. managed care's 'devil' of individual physicians. They are liable to gross error in assessing strength of real enemies, and they imagine themselves to be all-powerful experiencing a vast inflation of narcissism.

Change in personality of individuals caught-up in a mass movement may take place with lightning speed. To be able to trust the mass movement's contradictory, often absurd promises, requires a "missive regression" to a childish belief in omnipotence of the mass in conjunction with an intense identification of members of the mass with one another. Only strength of individual ego can prevail against attractions of such mass excitement; that, in fact, hope lies in fostering

---

[35] A.S. Relman. "Reforming the Health Care System." *New England Journal of Medicine* 323 (1990) 991-992.

[36] Lynn Etheredge, Stanley B. Jones, and Lawrence Lewin. "What Is Driving Health System Change?" *Health Affairs* 15 Winter (1996) 93-104.

[37] Sigmund Freud. *Group Psychology and the Analysis of the Ego.* 1921, p. 672.

development of the individual, that strength of individual ego is indissolubly bound up with ability to be critical of claims made by promoters, and with ability to resist overwhelming emotion and to distinguish between self and mass.[38] Promoters of managed care provoked emotions of fear and excitement, offered a chance of a lifetime, something for nothing, a glorious vision of the future, to conform by coercion.

A movement is taking place in the academic institutions and universities of America similar to the phenomenon of the managed care mass movement: an anti-intellectual, subjective appeal to irrationality denouncing Western science.[39] Almost any illogical statement can be made in the name of the supposed change in the "paradigm" of medical practice based on the theory of Thomas Kuhn, published in 1962. An anthropologist says, "The hapless Tom Kuhn (who is horrified by this particular mangling of his theory of paradigms)...[is] invoked like gods to justify an ultimately totally relativistic epistemology..."[40] i.e., a purely subjective claim that begs the question, and goes about to prove its insupportable claims, such as the desirability and inevitability of the managed care mass movement.

The powerful can be as timid as the weak when confronted by a mass movement; more important than power is faith in the future of the mass movement. To transform a nation, the movement must do so by breeding and captaining discontent or demonstrating desirability of change. Those with outstanding achievement, with full, happy lives tend to be against drastic change. Desire for a substitute for current circumstances is a craving for a new life, a rebirth, a chance to acquire new elements of pride, confidence, hope, a sense of purpose and worth by identifying with a holy cause: a mass movement offers such opportunities.[41]

Sir Thomas Browne, seventeenth-century British physician and author of *Religio Medici*, said, "The ears of the Vulgar [common people] are opener to Rhetorick than Logick," which allowed the hyperbole of the managed care industry to excite the mass movement into managed care. Charlatanism of some degree is indispensable to effective leadership in a mass movement, which requires deliberate misrepresentation of facts.[42]

---

[38] Alexander Mitscherlich. "Group Psychology and the Analysis of the Ego—A Lifetime Later." *Psychoanalytic Quarterly* (1978) 1-23.
[39] Robin Fox. "State of the Art/Science in Anthropology." in *The Flight From Science and Reason.* Paul R. Gross, Norman Levitt, & Martin W. Lewis, editors. *Annals of New York Academy of Science.* vol. 775. 1996, p. 335.
[40] Fox. p. 335.
[41] Hoffer. pp. 18-21.
[42] Hoffer. p. 107.

Like managed care, banking manias and financial panics are also associated with general irrationality, or mob psychology, but the relationship between rational individuals and irrational whole is complex: people will change at different stages of a continuing process, starting rationally and, gradually then more quickly, losing contact with reality. Rational behavior differs among groups of traders, investors, or speculators including those at earlier stages and those at later stages; all succumb to the *fallacy of composition*, which asserts that from time to time the whole is other than the sum of its parts.[43] Similar to the irrational mania of managed care, when caught in mass psychology of the eighteenth-century South Sea Bubble, a banker exclaimed, "When the rest of the world are mad, we must imitate them in some measure."[44]

---

[43] Kindleberger. pp. 23-24.
[44] Kindleberger. p. 24.

Chapter VI

THE BIND

VI. 1. CAPTIVITY

No choice—loss of identity—caught in a mass movement—sinking morale—captives—the bind.

The bind was expressed in rhetoric of captivity: "they've got us," "prisoners of insurance companies," "no way to turn," "no options," "there is no way to fight it." Even those physicians who might have resisted did not because it was too costly to fight the managed care industry and too few to have an effect. Employers were advised to "seek to divide the provider community" of physicians and hospitals into competing economic units or closed-panel groups of physicians.[1] Business adopted and supported divisive tactics of managed care advocates. Managed care attempted to control costs by modifying practices of doctors in various ways.[2]

The bind created the same feelings in physicians as seen in people in similar conflicts where individuals lose control, self-esteem, and identity when in captivity. Physicians expressed feelings of panic and powerlessness with their authority and integrity supplanted by the perceived power of the managed care industry, which held influence over health care. Physicians had difficulty dealing with the respectful way that patients still regarded them in contrast to what managed care plans were saying, that inside doctors felt demeaned. Physicians

---

[1] A.C. Enthoven and R. Kronick. "Competition 101: Managing Demand to get Quality Care." *Business and Health*. March 7 (1988) 38-40.

[2] A.S. Relman. "Controlling Costs by 'Managed Competition'—Would It Work?" *New England Journal of Medicine* 328 (1993) 133-135.

became an angry, demoralized profession feeling confused and threatened—hardly in the best interest of patient care.[3]

Managed care companies found they could alter physicians' practices by intimidation and coercion[4] using financial "incentives" to influence physicians' clinical decisions. Physicians and patients responded to what was in their own financial interests raising a crucial question as to whether financial incentives affected physicians' decisions and whether financial incentives distorted physicians' judgment. About two thirds of managed care plans that used a 'withhold' of a portion of the providers payment invoked penalties more severe than sacrificing their withhold account, for example, placing a lien on primary care physicians' future payments. The financial arrangement that received the most attention and concern was when managed care plans placed physicians at risk to lose their withheld income solely on the basis of budgetary outcome of their patients. By pressuring doctors to see more patients a day for a capitated fee itself increased costs, because doctors found the quickest way to terminate an office visit was to write a prescription rather than take time for explanation.[5] At the same time, honest and ethical doctors do not knowingly and willingly place their own financial self-interest above patients' best medical interests. When placed in a bind where the doctor must choose between limiting care and self-preservation produced a conflict that was not easily resolved.[6]

Concerns expressed about rationing of medical care by physicians were raised by policy makers who carefully avoided the word "rationing" by substituting emphasis on "beneficial services," or societal considerations beyond individual patients. Choosing a less expensive alternative on overall social benefit linked individual decisions to broader issues by saving in one instance to support costs in another was less persuasive when savings became profits to managed care companies. Appealing to "standard of care" may have been reasonable so long as the standard of care was reliable, good medical practice. If standard of care meant restricting reasonable care for profits, appealing to standard of care was not defensible. Displacing responsibility, or a compromise, to an external rule or authority or the requirements of a managed care company out of physicians' control eased doctors' consciences for a while; but physicians had to consider

[3] David R. Olmos and Michael A. Hiltzik. "Doctor's Authority, Pay Dwindle Under HMOs." *Los Angeles Times*. Aug 29, 1995.

[4] J.E. Kralewskyi, B. Dowd, R. Feldman, J. Shapiro. "The Physician Rebellion." *New England Journal of Medicine* 316 (1987) 339-342.

[5] Ron Winslow. "Health-Care Inflation Revives in Minneapolis Despite Cost-Cutting." *Wall Street Journal* May 19, 1998.

[6] Alan L. Hillman. "Health Maintenance Organizations, Financial Incentives, and Physicians Judgments." *Annals of Internal Medicine*. 112 (1990) 891-893.

effects of compromise, underlying motivations of those imposing constraints, and extent that physician's traditional and legal position was jeopardized. Physicians have strong and historic obligations to individual patients, but physicians cannot fight every battle forever.

Making do with less than the best created a bind where doctors were obliged to decide whether to provide good care or the best possible care. Such practice is a timeless and reasonable medical practice, however it became a bind if the doctor changed his practice after a managed care plan introduced financial incentives and penalties towards a less expensive approach to treatment. The goal was to practice medicine more effectively when compromise was inevitable.[7] Yet, physicians cannot serve patients as trusted counselors and agents with economic ties to the managed care industry that regards patients as customers.[8]

Managed care companies compelled physicians to sign "no cause" nonrenewal clauses in which their contracts could be terminated for any reason or no reason. Some managed care plans forbade doctors from telling patients what medical services the plan did and did not provide; and other similar restraints. Physicians under these restrictions became torn between their obligation to patients and obligation to their families, because with one or two expensive cases they could be dropped by a managed care plan. Such divided loyalties can be wrenching, because physicians were so threatened to keep their livelihood that they might no longer be willing to act as patients' advocates. So intense was intimidation that conscientious physicians at times became unwilling to advocate for patients even when they thought that a managed care plan had restricted care inappropriately. Physicians placed in this bind could not tolerate it, and that produced a greater threat—loss of integrity. Physicians found themselves obligated to conform to restrictions of managed care companies and deceived themselves that it was best for patients.[9] It was difficult if not impossible to practice ethical medicine in an unethical system.[10]

Prior to 1989, disability insurance companies considered doctors excellent insurance risks. About 80 percent of physicians had disability insurance; thirty percent of the in-force disability policies of many carriers were held by doctors. Today, many insurance companies no longer write disability policies for physicians, and if written, only at greatly increased premiums because more

---

[7] David A. Asch and Peter A. Ubel. "Rationing by Any Other Name." *New England Journal of Medicine* 336 (1997) 1668-1671.

[8] A.S. Relman. "Practicing Medicine in the New Business Climate." *New England Journal of Medicine* 316 (1987) 1150-1151.

[9] J.P. Kassirer. "Preserving Our Noble Heritage." *Western Journal of Medicine*. 164 (1996) 535-536.

[10] Erich H. Loewy. "Guidelines, Managed Care, and Ethics." *Archives of Internal Medicine* 156 (1996) 2038-2040.

physicians are receiving benefits and disability benefits longer than anticipated, but the main reason is a growing number of claims. Job satisfaction became as important as health problems: when individuals are satisfied with their work, less time is taken from work and recovery time is shorter. Managed care specifically impacted physicians and dentists. The safety net of disability insurance was no longer affordable; the honor and integrity that earned physicians most favored customer status with disability insurance companies no longer applied.[11]

Doctors were said to be the "officer corps" of our own health-care army, yet physician morale suffered since they were overwhelmed with insults and bureaucratic hassles by hundreds of managed care companies. Some doctors were greedy, but most made low to reasonable incomes doing one of the hardest job in the world, and the one requiring the most training yet experiencing low morale.[12] No wonder morale of practicing physicians and enthusiasm of young people for careers in medicine flagged. Physicians expected to be well paid for their efforts, although more personal rewards are also important.[13]

With hospitals in Southern California losing money, managed care plan managers had a new power, direct and implied, to dictate rates and treatment policies; hospitals lost managed care contracts by being patient advocates. Contracts were for one or two years, but they could be terminated by a managed care plan in 30 to 60 days during which payments to hospitals were sometimes drastically reduced. Although not many contracts were actually canceled, the bind created fear and warned rebellious physicians and hospitals.[14] The public was also in a bind, since many people were captives of the managed care industry in that enrollment of workers in managed care plans was dictated by employers and of Medicaid recipients by state governments, as well as Medicare by the federal government making managed care the only choice or only possible economic choice.[15]

The captive who led a quiet existence up to the time of captivity, is suddenly subjected to unbearable stress and hopelessness. The victim suffers a number of physical and emotional effects, and loved ones suffer by extension of the victim's

---

[11] Robert M. Terney, Jr. "Disability insurers no longer seek out physicians." *American Medical News* May 5, 1997.

[12] Melvin Konner. "We Are Not the Enemy: A Medical Opinion." *Newsweek* April 5, 1993; Joseph S. Alpert. "Where Have All the Flowers Gone: Where is the Joy in Medicine?" *Archives of Internal Medicine* 158 (1998) 693.

[13] A.S. Relman. "Shattuck Lecture—The Health Care Industry: Where is it Taking Us?" *New England Journal of Medicine* 325 (1991) 854-859.

[14] Erik Larson. "The Soul of an HMO." *Time* Jan. 22, 1996. 45-52.

[15] Thomas Bodenheimer. "The HMO Backlash—Righteous or Reactionary?" *New England Journal of Medicine* 335 (1996) 1601-1604.

trauma into their lives.[16] Hopelessness refers to a psychological characteristic of pessimism or negative expectancy; partially linked to affective disorders, depression, and to suicide intent.[17] A number of theories applied, such as the "systemic disaffection theory" with causal factors of perception of sociopolitical reality. The perceived threat to and/or loss of freedom is particularly important if the individual feels susceptible to such a threat or loss of freedom, or views himself as being comparable to others who have experienced such a threat or loss of freedom.

Herman Melville expresses the conflict of the individual versus the mass movement of managed care: "take mankind in mass, and, for the most part, they seem a mob of unnecessary duplicates, both contemporary and hereditary. But from the same point, take high abstracted man alone; and he seems a wonder, a grandeur, and a woe."[18] To physicians, patients possess a grandeur, but to the burkers of the managed care industry, a patient became an unnecessary duplicate, dehumanized "covered-life."

VI. 2. BEHAVIOR OF PHYSICIANS

Prior to advent of managed care, medical practice was carried on in a spirit of cooperation among colleagues, but managed care pitted doctors against one another. Physicians were rewarded for denying care depending on one's "ideological interpretation" implying that physicians were placed in a conflict.[19] By forming into groups, doctors became more controllable. With tens of thousands of doctors, no politician could hope to control that many individuals. Physicians quietly transformed from an arrogant independence to quiet subservience.

Given the character, personality make-up, and personal needs of physicians, how do we behave under stress? No one phenomenon accounts for the reaction of physicians to advance and threat of the managed care industry nor are these the only explanations possible. In addition, physicians are a diverse and varied group of individuals whose individualism has characterized the profession for centuries.

---

[16] Frank M. Ochberg and David A. Soskis. "Victims of Terrorism." *Westview Special Studies in National and International Terrorism.* Boulder, Colo.: Westview Press, 1982. pp. vii, 30-31.

[17] R.R. Holden. "Hopelessness." *Encyclopedia of Psychology* Editor Raymond J. Corsini. 2nd edition. Vol. 2. New York: John Wiley & Sons, 1994, p. 156.

[18] Herman Melville. *Moby-Dick or The Whale* (1861) Evanston and Chicago: Northwestern University Press, 1988. p. 466.

[19] Laura Mechler. "Higher co-payments keep HMO premiums down." *San Francisco Examiner* May 4, 1997.

We react in diverse and varied ways. Not surprising, then, physicians responded as do other groups who are placed in a bind or captivity. Physicians were intimidated into thinking that we must participate as a matter of professional and economic survival. In studies of prisoners faced with deprivation, torture, and threats of death, many prisoners become detached, emotionless, and indifferent to events taking place around them.[20] The captive is deliberately, unjustly harmed or coerced by another human being, feels diminished, pushed down in a hierarchy of dominance, exploited, and invaded.[21] The silence of physicians was a puzzling phenomenon, which arose at least in part from a feeling of captivity.

The bind was heightened by unjust accusations of intentional and excessive utilization of resources; variations in practice patterns occur because good doctors often disagree resulting in variations in practice from doctor to doctor, hospital to hospital, and city to city. Managed care companies placed restrictions on physicians to a range of options that reflected management decisions. Variations from practice guidelines led to sanctions against doctors for non-compliance, from non-payment to termination of privileges. Financial incentives made physicians responsible for both patients' clinical interests and the organization's financial solvency, a dual mandate: treat the patient, but within budget so managed care organizations prosper. Physicians as agents of management conflicts with physicians' traditional role. In contrast, courts consistently affirm physicians' responsibility to uphold standards of care for individual patients independent of rules and incentives.[22]

Psychologists regard physicians as narcissistic with many ego needs that are both our trait and our strength because the work we do requires doctors to have a favorable opinion of who we are and what we do. The *narcissist-under-stress* is another matter, risking major depressions and volatile eruptions of anger. A passive, dejected lethargy may occur when narcissists experience threats to their egos. Ego and narcissism drive any successful professional far more than the 'bottom line.'[23]

Though physicians are individualistic, we are also members of a group, and, to a certain extent, behave as other groups. Groups, like individuals, appear to be motivated not only by overt aims, but also by tensions arising out of unconscious aims, conflicts, and defenses. Formal organizations coerce individuals to suppress

---

[20] Atkinson, Atkinson, and Hilgard. *Introduction to Psychology.* Eighth Edition. Chapt. 14 "Conflict and Stress." New York: Harcourt Brace Jovanovich, 1983, pp. 426-431.

[21] Frank M. Ochberg. "Post-Traumatic Therapy and Victims of Violence.' in *Post-Traumatic Therapy and Victims of Violence.* Editor Frank M. Ochberg. New York: Brunner/Mazel, 1988, pp. 3-81.

[22] Alan L. Hillman. "Managing The Physician: Rules Versus Incentives." *Health Affairs* 10 Winter (1991) 138-146.

[23] Donald Trump. "What My Ego Wants, My Ego Gets." *New York Times* Sep 17, 1995.

internal conflict, limit interpersonal conflict, and control expression of emotion in order to concentrate energies and attention on purposes of the group. To accomplish aims of the group requires a shared culture, a shared myth or ideology—as part of regressive features of this myth or ideology, the exercise of power becomes an expression of that myth. Those persons who try to maintain individuality are targets for attack. Simplistic generalizations or ideologies are eagerly received—"embraced"—and have a calming effect.[24]

The surrender of physicians and medical community, as well as the public, into managed care with little protest also conformed to a mass or crowd psychological phenomenon in two fundamental features of crowds' effect upon individuals: regression and merging of individual identity with that of the crowd. Deliberation gives way to impulsiveness. Suggestibility and imitation determine decisions at the expense of moral and rational considerations. In diversity of a crowd, unconscious foundations of the mind, instincts common to all members of a crowd, are intensified and exert a greater influence. Thus, exaggerated feelings of helplessness coincided with frustration of dependent wishes to "embrace" managed care.[25]

The *Stockholm syndrome*, a bond between captive and captor with negative feelings toward society, explains the readiness of some physicians to embrace managed care without effort, forethought or resistance. Physicians experienced denial that such a phenomenon could possibly take place. Denial in the captive gives way to delusions of reprieve, that by embracing managed care, the managed care industry would look after them. The Stockholm Syndrome is an automatic, often unconscious, emotional response to trauma of being a victim—the victim's need to survive is stronger than his impulse to hate the captor, and a way to relieve stress caused by loss of independence. Most people cannot inflict pain or distress on another person unless the victim is *dehumanized*—a *corollary* to the Stockholm syndrome. The patient was no longer an individual, but became declassified from a patient into a 'covered life' which made mistreatment less offensive and more tolerable.

A state of *cognitive dissonance* may occur if we have few choices. Doctors who were well compensated accepted managed care schemes with little attitude change and little dissonance. When low paid physicians joined managed care

---

[24] Burness E. Moore and Kenneth T. Calder. "Psychoanalytic Knowledge of Group Processes." *Journal of the American Psychoanalytic Association* 27 (1979) 145-156.
[25] Stephen M. Saravay. "Group Psychology and the Structural Theory: A Revised Psychoanalytic Model of Group Psychology." *Journal of the American Psychoanalytic Association* 23 (1975) 69-89.

plans, they experienced distress and dissonance, which was relieved by experiencing an attitude change in order to relieve their distress.

Fear provoking metaphors led to relieving the bind by concluding, or being convinced, that there were no alternatives, a *death march,* when all avenues of reprieve have been exhausted. A one-sided argument led many to think that to resist or search for alternatives to managed care was futile; anxiety was relieved.

Although doctors initially most eager for managed care were primary care doctors, the most staunch opponents were also a few primary care doctors who refused to participate in managed care plans. After experience with managed care, many physicians discovered they were deceived, and their conversion to managed care did not relieve their distress and anxiety for long. The solution offered by managed care promoters was to "go wholly into managed care" and "make it work." But, doctors came to see that managers of managed care, and managed care companies profited at their expense.

In negotiating with managed care companies, physicians felt especially vulnerable. For a negotiation to be fair or equitable, each side or player must have an equal chance of winning a contested, reasonable point. Mathematicians speak of *game theory* of negotiation, and players must decide whether the game they are in is played fairly. The 'withhold' of twenty percent or more of payments to physicians by managed care companies illustrates distortion of the game. Since the doctor had little or no chance in negotiating with a managed care company, the game was rigged. The 'withhold' became an *inducement,* or *entrapment.*

The *prisoner's dilemma* comes close to the present situation in managed care. In this instance, each of two prisoners occupying the same cell is separately offered $1,000 or $3,000 to the other prisoner. In nearly every instance, the individual acts selfishly and accepts the $1,000 rather than larger amount to share with the other prisoner. In this 'non-cooperative game,' prisoner and physician act selfishly which theorists say occurs in nearly every case in non-cooperative games.

In the *Nash Equilibrium* of game theory, one player is risk-averse and will avoid risk at all costs; the other is risk-neutral and will take a reasonable risk if necessary. In this case, the risk averse-player will tend to settle for less than the risk-neutral player whether the two are allowed to communicate or negotiate with each other in a 'cooperative game,' or whether they act independently without communication. Physicians and physician groups acted in a risk-averse manner assuming that they were playing it safe by accepting 'at risk' contracts or face 'revenue lock-out,' but had little or no chance of winning in these negotiations. The Nash Equilibrium is based on a combination of strategies that players may choose in which no player can do better with a different strategy given the strategies of the other players. By asking whether either player has an incentive to deviate from equilibrium establishes whether a strategy combination is in fact a Nash Equilibrium. In the case of the managed care mass movement, physicians and other providers do have an incentive to deviate from the strategy of the managed care industry, consequently, no Nash Equilibrium exists.[26]

Physician behavior, then, is understandable when put in a conflict, a bind. Since physicians were forbidden to bargain collectively with managed care companies, physicians were forced into a non-cooperative game—each physician must decide which choice he or she would make. The bind was not easily resolved or dismissed. Physicians' personal gain also influences practice patterns, including non-financial gains, such as practicing in a certain environment and achieving intellectual or professional satisfaction. Dealing with uncertainty in medical practice with the goal of achieving certainty can lead to over-testing; professional instinct attributes greater seriousness to errors of omission than to errors of commission. Uncertainty leads to greater use of resources; it does not mean unacceptable practice. The range of acceptable practice is broad enough to allow substantial variations. Even major differences in hospitalization or surgical rates do not necessarily indicate good or bad practices, only different practices.[27]

Managed care organizations were also based on uncertainty. The goal was to reduce health care costs by reducing access to or use of resources by several methods: regulating or controlling practices by utilization review and sanctions against physicians, altering physician behavior by financial incentives or medical practice guidelines. If conservation incentive was so strong as to cause under-utilization by not providing necessary care, unacceptable care resulted. Both practicing physicians and managed care companies operated on the same continuum of uncertainty: from under utilization, through appropriate utilization, to excessive utilization. Differences in incentives and other personal, professional, or organizational objectives drove each toward one end of the spectrum or the other. Uncertainty prompted managed care companies to restrict access to save money claiming that what was not known for certain was inappropriate care, i.e. the error of *argumentum ad ignorantiam*. Physicians claimed that ethical responsibility and obligation to patients derives from history, culture, and law, and that only regularly practicing physicians can determine acceptable utilization

---

[26] Douglas G. Baird, Robert H. Gertner, and Randal C. Picker. *Game Theory and the Law.* Cambridge, Mass and London: Harvard University Press, 1994, pp. 19-24, 310; R.J. Aumann. "Game Theory" in *Game Theory* editors John Eatwell, Murray Milgate, and Peter Newman. New York and London: W.W. Norton, 1989, pp. 1-53.
[27] David M. Mirvis and Cyril F. Chang. "Managed Care, Managing Uncertainty." *Archive of Internal Medicine* 157 (1997) 385-388.

which entails uncertainty in clinical practice, since only professional judgment and experience can effectively decide what should or should not be done in the absence of absolute knowledge.[28]

The image persists of a doctor as a benevolent, knowledgeable being whose principal aim was to make patients well, and that critics don't give doctors much credit for pride, ethics, practicality and love for their profession.[29] Although many see managed care as an abstract dilemma, increasingly the struggle became more concrete and stark: physicians forced to choose between best interests of patients and economic survival. Doctors forced into a bind find themselves conforming to managed care restrictions and deceiving themselves that what they are doing is best for their patients.[30] The passivity of physicians, in some measure, allowed the profession of medicine to be subsumed into the managed care mass movement.

As early as 1983, a fundamental weakness of managed care was recognized that it was based on an uncritical application of the concept of incentives: "That policy should 'change the incentives' to bring behavior into line with what government seeks has the ring of unassailable insight, eternal truth, elegant simplicity." Incentives may be capable of doing some things to some degree and others very little or not at all; little was known what problems were amenable to what types of incentive-based solutions.[31]

Unification in managed care by doctors and patients was more a diminution than of addition, being stripped of free choice and independent judgment. The adherent in a mass movement is forever incomplete and insecure.[32] In a mass movement, the adherent is convinced that the cause is eternal, and a sense of security is derived from the perceived excellence of the cause—not so much by the principles of the cause, but because of the adherent's need for something to hold on to, and cannot be separated from the cause by reason or moral sense.[33] Mass sentiments and acts are contagious: individuals readily sacrifice personal interest to collective interest which is contrary to their nature except when part of a mass as if hypnotized, and they will accomplish acts of irresistible impetuosity

---

[28] Mirvis and Chang.
[29] Louise Kertesz. "Root of all evil?" *Modern Healthcare* Mar 17, 1997.
[30] J.P. Kassirer. "Managed Care and the Marketplace." *New England Journal of Medicine* 333 (1995) 50-52.
[31] Lawrence D. Brown. *Politics and Health Care Organization: HMOs as Federal Policy.* Washington, DC: The Brookings Institution, 1983, p. 449.
[32] Eric Hoffer. *The True Believer.* New York: Harper & Row, 1951. p. 117.
[33] Hoffer. pp. 80-81,

and gain strength by reciprocity. Those who might resist are too few to struggle against the current.[34]

VI. 3. BEATING THE SCHEME

Business and individual purchasers of managed care plans appeared willing to take a chance that somehow they could beat the odds, or work the system. Doctors who "embraced" managed care disregarded cautions and warnings about risks of managed care. Where managed care was taking us was not clear, but some claimed that independent office medical practice was not likely to continue. Whether doctors in managed care would be able to maintain influence and autonomy as advocates for their patients remained to be seen, and that doctors would have to re-dedicate themselves to traditional ethics of medicine, that doctors would have to work together which was forbidden by law.[35]

Generalists, family practitioners, hailed the revolution and decried specialization with return to non-specialist emphasis in medical practice, and took satisfaction that the era of specialist-technologists had passed. Yet, generalists who assumed the role of gate-keeper in managed care gained experience that their lot in practice did not improve as many anticipated, and in some respects were worse because they had greater responsibility as well as liability.[36] Many physicians seemed busy to the point of frenzy, complaining about working harder and harder to barely keep pace with exploding size of office staffs to keep up with managed care paperwork. At first, some believed they were working together to curb the "abuses and excesses" of traditional fee-for-service practice, but managed care plans' demands cured their naiveté.[37]

Efforts to gain control of physicians and practice of medicine by the managed care industry with sanction of business and government succeeded in rapid growth of managed care. "Go wholly into managed care" and all problems of delivery and costs would be solved with a promise of a vague, glorious future.

---

[34] Gustave Le Bon. *The Crowd: A Study of the Popular Mind.* (1895) Dunwoody, GA: Norman S. Berg, 2nd ed. 1984, pp. 10-12.

[35] A.S. Relman. "The Changing Climate of Medical Practice. Introduction." *New England Journal of Medicine* 316 (1987) 333-334.

[36] Richard L. Garrison. "The Five Generations of American Medical Revolutions." *Journal of Family Practice* 40 (1995) 281-287.

[37] Philip R. Alper. "Managed care, too, shall pass–the sooner the better." *Medical Economics* 17 June (1991) 93-96.

VI. 4. Some Legal Aspects of Managed Care

The relationship between physician and patient, the basis of any health care delivery system, is immensely complex. Because a patient depends upon a physician in time of need and cannot fully assess quality of service delivered, the relationship is intrinsically asymmetric with physicians assuming extraordinary trust from patients and are expected to take a fiduciary role. The physician-patient relationship assumes not only therapeutic and humanitarian values, but also carries legal and ethical implications.[38]

The physician-patient relationship underwent a dramatic change under managed care in that decisions doctors and patients made jointly were limited by managed care companies which were influenced by factors out of physicians' control: operation of the managed care plan, its gatekeeping rules, attitude of its agents and employees, etc.[39] Physicians' primary legal duty was to patients, not to managed care plans, and not altered by participation in managed care.[40] The physician is obligated to protest and intercede in behalf of patients, stated by a California court: "While we recognize, realistically, that cost consciousness has become a permanent feature of the health care system, it is essential that cost limitation programs not be permitted to corrupt medical judgment."[41] Health plans could be held legally accountable when medically inappropriate decisions resulted from cost containment mechanisms, for example, when appeals made on patients' behalf for medical or hospital care were arbitrarily ignored, unreasonably disregarded, or overridden. However, physicians who complied without protest with limitations imposed by a third-party payer when physician's medical judgment dictated otherwise cannot avoid responsibility for the outcome of a patient's care.[42]

The 'gatekeeper,' with a significant role in managed care and some prestige, assumed a new liability. Even if a primary care physician referred the patient to a specialist and the specialist recommended additional consultation, the patient must

---

[38] David M. Mirvis. "Doctor-Patient and Doctor-Patient-Society Relationships after Health Care Reform." in *Beyond the Crisis: Preserving the Capacity for Excellence in Health Care and Medical Science* Henry M. Greenberg and Susan U. Raymond, editors. *Annals of the New York Academy of Sciences* 729, 1994, pp. 55-61.

[39] David Karp. "Managed Care Liability: What Physicians Should Consider." *Loss Minimizer* Nov. 1993.

[40] Philip R. Hinderberger. "Re: Senate Judiciary Committee Hearing Regarding 'Potential Issues of Antitrust, Unfair Competition, Fair Bargaining and Contracts, Liability Arising from Negligent or Unavailable Care, and Other Issues Raised by the Use of Capitation Agreements for the Delivery of Professional Medical Care." June 6, 1995.

[41] Karp.

[42] Karp.

return to the primary care physician for care that would normally be carried out by a specialist. Each of these added duties assumed added liability. Primary care physicians were also at risk under utilization review if the number of hospitalizations was considered too great, lengths of stay too long, or if number of referrals to specialists was deemed excessive by a managed care company. A variety of pressures were applied to primary care physicians to correct "costly practices," so that primary care physician's medical judgment could not avoid giving way to cost considerations. The primary care doctor was held to the standard of care of a specialist by statute if patients were not referred to appropriate specialists.

Primary care doctors who were gatekeepers assumed greatest potential liability because of the bind: if they protested too hard and too often, they risked being dropped from managed care plans. If managed care contracts contained financial incentives like capitation and withholds that discouraged particular treatments, those incentives could be used against doctors to convince jurors that the doctor put personal interests ahead of patients' medical needs.[43] Non-solicitation clauses, or 'gag-orders,' restricted physicians from expressing negative views of managed care plans to patients, or from advising patients regarding selection of managed care plans. Managed care plans contended that the provision was necessary to prevent doctors from shifting patients into other plans. Gag orders were considered "morally suspect." The First Constitutional Amendment and right to free speech was abridged by the managed care industry.[44]

In response to legal complications of contracts with managed care plans, new legislation was introduced and a few laws were enacted in California: elimination of the gag clause; requiring managed care plans to disclose types of physician reimbursement to enrollees and prohibit certain physician incentive plans; and the right of patients to an independent medical review outside of their managed care plan when their plan intended to deny coverage for treatment that was experimental or investigational.[45] Medical ethicists were concerned that managed care plans improperly intruded into private physician-patient conversations. Physicians saw that non-solicitation clauses forced doctors to give up First Amendment free speech rights in exchange for being a member of a managed care

---

[43] Berkeley Rice. "Look who's on the malpractice hot seat now: But don't think doctors are off the hook." *Medical Economics.* Aug 12 (1996) 193-205.

[44] "Background Paper for Capitation Hearing." California Legislature, Senate Committee on Judiciary. 6 June 1995.

[45] *Capital Pulse.* California Medical Association. Dec. 1996.

company's provider group. Patients were denied important information about deficiencies in managed care plans.[46]

"Hold harmless clauses," particularly onerous to physicians, stipulated that managed care plans and physicians shall "hold each other harmless" from costs associated with activities governed by their contracts. This clause, in effect, restricted doctors from suing the managed care plan's provider group when the doctor adhered to a managed care plan's decision and resulted in medical liability. Hold harmless and indemnification clauses bind physicians to pay settlements and judgments plus legal costs in liability cases in which managed care organizations were named as a defendant. Some managed care agreements required physicians to hold the managed care organization harmless from all liability for a managed care organization's decision to deny benefits to patients.[47] Hold harmless clauses were deemed essential by managed care plans in light of Wickline vs. State of California (1986), which held that a third party payer may be liable in damages for injury suffered by utilization or managed care decisions.[48]

Managed care companies knew there was almost no money for plaintiff attorneys in litigating in favor of patients against managed care companies. Plaintiffs' attorneys exchanged strategies and information on how to broaden the range of defendants to include outside firms such as those providing utilization review, writing practice guidelines, accrediting agencies, credentialing organizations, and especially employers who contract with or sponsor managed care plans. Some members of the insurance industry have said that the same legal principles used against managed care companies could be applied to employers. In order to protect themselves, many employers demanded that managed care contracts protect them from joint liability claims.[49] In order to protect themselves from liability arising from vicarious liability tort actions, managed care companies used broad indemnification agreements in provider contracts to pass their liability on to physicians and hospitals.[50] Conferences provided counsel to managed care plans on how managed care plans could structure their physician contracts to avoid or minimize legal liability by diverting the entire liability to physicians, hospitals, and other medical providers. Managed care companies found they were

---

[46] "Background Paper for Capitation Hearing." California Legislature. Senate Committee on Judiciary. Senator Charles M. Calderon, Chairman.

[47] Karp.

[48] "Background Paper for Capitation Hearing." California Legislature. Senate Committee on Judiciary. Senator Charles M. Calderon, Chairman.

[49] Rice.

[50] Hinderberger.

vulnerable to liability from legislative action of 'single-issue bills' from outpatient mastectomies to sweeping federal legislation.[51]

When managed care plans were sued, plans sought protection behind a provision of Employee Retirement Income Security Act of 1974, called ERISA, which covers nearly three-quarters of all people who receive health insurance through their employers. Patients could sue ERISA-covered managed care plans, but only in federal court where plaintiffs' burden of proof was much greater than in state courts. Even if successful, plaintiffs could recover only cost of benefits denied, but not for lost wages, physical injury or other claims. Plaintiffs' lawyers contended that ERISA enabled managed care plans to deny patients' access to treatment without risk of legal liability, and medical organizations claimed that ERISA unfairly placed excessive liability on physicians as a result of the decisions of managed care plans. Until recently, managed care companies have successfully defended against most liability claims by citing ERISA pre-emption. Some cases claimed that managed care companies were "vicariously liable" for quality of care rendered by their physicians and were "ostensible agents" of managed care companies. Managed care companies had thought that ERISA would effectively shield health plans from liability, although several large judgments against managed care companies have been awarded.[52]

Due to ERISA law, business was protected from liability for restrictive practices of managed care plans, which was a mute condoning of managed care industry methods: who wills the ends wills the means. Congress could overturn exemption of employer-sponsored health plans that cover as estimated 140 million Americans and 60% of families. Passed into law in 1974, ERISA was never intended to be a liability barrier for health plans, and courts chipped away at ERISA.[53] ERISA law acquired a second life as a way that managed care could avoid state-court jurisdiction when members brought suit. Managed care plans insisted that suits against them be transferred to federal court. Once in federal court, judges generally ruled that pension law exempted both corporate employers and health plans from being liable for negligence.[54] It may be possible to circumvent ERISA if patients purchased their own insurance, but not if employers purchased insurance. The ERISA law "thwarts the legitimate claims of the very people it was designed to protect," who are left without meaningful remedy. The

---

[51] Wayne J. Guglielmo. "Roping down managed care." *Medical Economics*. June 23 (1997) 106-120.
[52] Rice.
[53] Geri Aston. "Making managed care share malpractice risks." *American Medical News* May 12, 1997.
[54] George Anders. *Health Against Wealth: HMOs and the Breakdown of Medical Trust*. Boston and New York: Houghton Mifflin, 1996. p. 255.

courts say that modifying the law must be done by Congress because the law is especially complex and detailed.[55] In addition, some managed care companies demanded physicians buy their liability insurance from an insurer selected by the managed care company, in some cases from an insurer owned by the managed care company itself.[56]

The managed care industry, following the lead of Kaiser *Permanente*, relied on arbitration to reduce its liability costs. Little information is available because results of Kaiser *Permanente* arbitration proceedings were closely guarded. A mandatory system of arbitration, which bars members from suing in court, could be dominated and manipulated by large managed care plans with the aim of obstructing fair settlements. After listening to a Kaiser *Permanente* member's story and Kaiser *Permanente's* defense, a Superior Court Judge declared Kaiser *Permanente's* arbitration system "'fraudulent,' 'unconscionable' and 'corrupt...in general.'"

A plaintiff's arbitrator in Kaiser *Permanente* liability cases said that he advised plaintiffs that it's very difficult to win against Kaiser *Permanente*, because patients must be prepared to spend $25,000 and upward for experts, saying that it's intended as a "stacked deck," and the unwary get caught. Although Kaiser *Permanente* attorneys claimed it wanted these cases over as quickly as possible, typical Kaiser *Permanente* arbitrations often took longer than similar cases in state court. In only 1 (one) percent of cases was a neutral arbitrator appointed within 60 days specified in the arbitration agreement, which on average took 667 days. Reaching a final resolution of arbitration took an average of 863 days. By comparison, getting a case to trial in the Oakland Appeals Court required only 15 to 19 months. Nevertheless, in 1992 Kaiser *Permanente* Health Plan paid $150 million in self-insured risks, primarily for professional liability.

Kaiser *Permanente* dominated the infrastructure of arbitration in that Kaiser *Permanente* was the largest single user of arbitration process in California. Kaiser *Permanente* kept close account on how arbitrators acted: if an arbitrator did not agree with Kaiser's attorneys, there was a good chance that arbitrator would not be chosen again. Patient advocates and consumer activists said that since arbitration is private and does not set legal precedent, arbitration tended to block access to information about the managed care industry. Thus, less could be learned about Kaiser *Permanente* and other managed care companies by the court system than about almost any other medical institution. People in managed care plans lost access to courts; consequently, a check on medical quality was also lost,

[55] Robert Pear. "Hands Tied, Judges Rue Law That Limits H.M.O. Liability." *New York Times* July 11, 1998. p. 1.
[56] Hinderberger.

which became more important in that patients gave up much of their freedom to choose their own doctors and hospitals in exchange for lower health insurance premiums with less opportunity to control their medical care.[57]

Anti-trust issues arose when current federal anti-trust laws, the Sherman Act and the Clayton Act, prohibited doctors from associating with other doctors to gain bargaining power against managed care companies dictating price and terms of health care in a market dominated by managed care plans. Without economic power, individual physicians were coerced by managed care plans to accept onerous contract terms that could impede doctors' ability to care for patients by controlling a significant segment of a doctor's patients.[58] Physicians were expected to exercise independent medical judgment when providing medical care to patients while at the same time expected to be a 'team player' when implementing managed care utilization management policies.[59] The obligation of physician to patients was stated clearly more than a century ago; in the case of Becker v. Janinski, in a New York Appellate Court in 1891.[60]

Costs of legal aspects of medical care were enormous; in 1994, 22% or $160 billion of total health care costs went to liability and defensive medicine.[61] As physicians and other health professionals became aware of a need to defend against professional liability suits, they were required to keep more extensive records which required more physician-time as well as time of office assistants, but this extra expense did not increase provision of professional services.[62] Certain features of managed care practice—notably, intensive scheduling and harried and resentful physicians—can lead to abrupt, impersonal care.[63]

In 1997, Connecticut approved a law granting patients and doctors outside review of a health plan's decision to deny care. Texas passed a landmark measure that allowed patients to sue managed care companies for malpractice, the first in the nation.[64] The managed care industry could not escape public scrutiny,

---

[57] Michael A. Hiltzik and David R. Olmos. "'Kaiser Justice' System's Fairness Questioned." *Los Angeles Times.* Aug 30, 1995.

[58] "Background Paper for Capitation Hearing." California Legislature. Senate Committee on Judiciary. Senator Charles M. Calderon, Chairman. June 6, 1995.

[59] Hinderberger.

[60] Hinderberger.

[61] Robert O'Brien. "The Doctor-Patient Relationship." in *Beyond the Crisis: Preserving the Capacity for Excellence in Health Care and Medical Science* Henry M. Greenberg and Susan U. Raymond, editors. *Annals of the New York Academy of Sciences* 729, 1994, pp. 22-26.

[62] Victor R. Fuchs. "The Health Sector's Share of the Gross National Product." *Science* 247 (1990) 534-538.

[63] Brown. p. 190.

[64] Susan Brink and Nancy Shute. "Managed care is pushing aside the private-practice doctors typified by TV's Marcus Welby or Dr. Kildare. What's replacing them isn't making anyone smile." *US. News and World Report* Oct. 13, 1997.

although greater regulation or legal restrictions were not likely to alter the course of mass movement into managed care.

The gathering criticism of the managed care industry produced a number of legislative initiatives in 1998 to curb abuses by managed care; the industry was willing to grant 'reforms' in order to preserve its immunity from liability by blocking patients' ability sue managed care plans.[65] However, a new development surfaced: courts in California allowed a charge of fraud against Cigna HealthCare for substituting a physician's assistant for an obstetrician instead of a claim of medical malpractice, which brought managed care fraud out of closed doors of arbitration into public view. Health Net and Secure Horizons drew the ire of patient advocacy groups for substituting a less expensive antidepressant medicine without knowledge of both patient and doctor.[66] In latter 1990s, courts across the country allowed more patients to sue managed care plans for malpractice and other legal principles gained support in Congress and the Administration. The Supreme Court of Pennsylvania concluded that the United States Supreme Court changed its stand in 1995 saying, "Congress did not intend to pre-empt state laws which govern the provision of safe medical care." Nevertheless, the complexity of federal and state law remained "in flux, often limited, and confusing" that would take time to clarify.[67]

VI. 5. MONEY. TRUST

In most societies, physicians have been well compensated. Adam Smith (1776) says: "[Public admiration] makes a considerable part of that reward in the profession of physic [medicine]."[68] He points out importance of responsibility of members of professions in the matter of trust: "Education [in professions such as medicine], is still more tedious and expensive. The pecuniary recompense, therefore, of...physicians, ought to be much more liberal: and it is so accordingly."[69] Smith's emphasis on trust of the public in the profession of medicine has modern significance: physicians' "reward must be such, therefore,

[65] Robert Pear. "H.M.O. Group Backs Controls G.O.P. Rejects." *New York Times*. July 14, 1998.

[66] Kristen Bole. "Consumer advocates give HMOs bitter pill to swallow." *San Francisco Business Times*. July 10-16, 1998. p. 11.

[67] Robert Pear. "Series of Rulings Eases Costratints on Suing H.M.O.'S: New Gains for Patients." *New York Times* August 15, 1999.

[68] Adam Smith. *An Inquiry into the Nature and Causes of The Wealth of Nations*. (1776) reprint. New York: The Modern Library, 1994. p 123.

[69] Adam Smith. p. 118.

as may give them that rank in the society which so important a trust requires."[70] A contemporary economist says that physicians lengthy period of education, long hours of work, absence of pensions, paid vacations, and other benefits accounts for the level of physicians' reimbursements.[71] Physicians under managed care, especially those who have taken positions of management and utilization review, were especially vulnerable to pressures of corporate medicine, and at risk to compromise physicians' responsibility and public trust. The necessary financial support of medicine blended with need for service, sacrifice, and trustworthiness in face of criticism.

The issue of cost of medical care was no longer absolute cost, rising costs or otherwise, but return from such expenditure, i.e. value or trust in the work of the profession of medicine.[72] The health care system will not work for patients unless it works for doctors.[73] According to an administrator of a major hospital, "No money, no mission."[74] The physician who abrogates trust by complicity with the managed care industry to the detriment of patient care, relinquishes qualifying for recompense due physicians by public trust.

Prior to the twentieth century, diagnosis and treatment created a bond between doctor and patient. The development of scientific medicine in late-nineteenth century was greeted by the public with a sense of awe. Scientific evidence eclipsed thoughts and feelings of patients who grew increasingly ambivalent; science shifted attention away from human concerns. Cultivation of trust during times of great change is difficult. Society holds medical doctors to a responsibility beyond that of a profession, beyond that of nearly all other professions—almost within the realm of supernatural belief; a patient brings a spiritual conviction about life and death for which no correlative in medical science exists. On the other hand, a businessperson is trusted to act ethically and with integrity, but also is expected to be motivated by economic self-interest—to sell as much goods and services as possible.[75]

[70] Adam Smith. pp. 118-123.

[71] V.R. Fuchs. *Essays in Economics of Health and Medical Care.* V.R. Fuchs, editor. New York and London: National Bureau of Economic Research, Columbia university Press, 1972, p. 48.

[72] David Thompson, James Harrison, and James Flanagan. "From paradigms lost to paradigms regained? The MILTON approach to health care reform." *Journal of Management in Medicine* (1995) 21-34.

[73] J.P. Kassirer. "Medicine at Center Stage." *New England Journal of Medicine* 328 (1993) 1268-1269.

[74] Mike O'Hara. "Managed Care: Is it good? Is it bad? Is it something in between?" *Mayo Alumni* Spring (1997) 8-13.

[75] Joseph P. Lyons. "The American Medical Doctor in the Current Milieu: A Matter of Trust." *Perspectives in Biology and Medicine.* 37 (1994) 443-459.

When vulnerable, an individual trusts and does not expect to be harmed, so that belief in another's good will goes unstated and understood. A trustworthy person cares, uses discretionary powers wisely and responsibly, neither excessively nor deficiently while giving assurances of trustworthiness.[76] The concept of trust in physician-patient relationships involves individual physicians and individual patients, not institutions that surround them.[77]

Patient trust has been perceived as falling to an "alarming low" in both Britain and United States. Most destructive to trust has been the "startling embrace" of belief that marketplace ethics and competition would improve medicine or make it less expensive, and in a profession where sensitivities of one's fellow man should be paramount, yet we are "absolutely bewildered" by how many physicians accepted a marketplace philosophy. Those who were basically trusting and permissive, and those who were distrustful and regulatory have conflicting concepts of reality, and viewed each other suspiciously.[78] New knowledge, increased education, and improved communication changed patients also; the spirit of the times was against authority.[79] Good medicine is and always has been based on mutual trust: trust that is earned, not given, and there are as many different ways of building trust as there are patients and doctors.[80]

The illusion of so-called wealth of physicians is more a public subconscious need than whether or not a doctor is financially solvent. Since less than one in ten doctors can be said to be "economically secure" leaves doubt that practice of medicine is the road to riches. Patients do not want his or her doctor to be more concerned about mortgage payments than their own best interests, which allows for conjuring the fancy that doctors are above ordinary cares. Those individuals in the profession of medicine and medical institutions may be well to follow biblical advice of having a crop laid-up, in addition to Samuel Johnson's advice to a friend about the cost of regaining his health: "Do not think about frugality, your health is worth more than it can cost."[81]

---

[76] Nancy Potter. "Discretionary Power, Lies, and Borken Trust: Justification and Discomfort." *Theoretical Medicine* 17 (1996) 329-352.

[77] Lee N. Newcomer. "Measures of Trust in Health Care." *Health Affairs* 16 (1997) 50-51.

[78] David E. Rogers. "On Trust: a basic building block for healing doctor-patient interactions." *Journal of the Royal Society of Medicine* 87 Suppl. 22(1994) 2-6.

[79] Joseph P. Horder. "The historical perspective." *Journal of the Royal Society of Medicine* 87 Suppl. 22 (1994) 6-8.

[80] Dame Margaret Turner-Warwick. "Paternalism versus patient autonomy." *Journal of the Royal Society of Medicine* 87 Suppl. 22 (1994) 16.

[81] R.W. Chapman. (ed.), *The Letters of Samuel Johnson*, 3 vols. Oxford: Clarendon Press, 1984, iii, 498-499. cited by Roy Porter. *Doctor of Society: Thomas Beddoes and the Sick Trade in Late-Enlightenment England* London and New York: Routledge, 1992, p. 124.

VI. 6. MEDICAL "INFLATION"

A system that increased average life span 28 years in less than a century entails a cost, which some have called "spiraling costs [in an] inflation-prone health industry." Physicians can be faulted for not informing the public that high quality, effective medical care is expensive.[82] Annual medical costs of seven major diseases account for about one-half of today's health care bill. The cost of bringing a single drug to market exceeds $350 million, which takes an average of 12 years.[83]

News media play a role in costs of medical care. Through the 1950s, 1960s, and 1970s, medical advances came so fast such that only "breakthroughs" were newsworthy. Hardly a week passed without a "breakthrough" excitedly reported in newspapers or on television. Hearing of startling new advances, patients sought new treatments or technological miracles. Reports of dramatic new therapies are often excessive, adding to public demand for medical services that doctors may consider ill advised. On occasion, news reporting brings important problems to public attention and into effective treatment.[84]

Despite more than a decade of cost-control efforts, Medicare costs were expected to grow more than 10 percent annually during latter part of the 1990s. Medicare Part B is expected to triple in cost by 2050. Many still assume that moving the elderly into managed care will cut costs without cutting benefits.[85] Neither managed care nor fee-for-service providers will be able to control long-term rise in costs except by rationing, i.e. denying some patients access to certain types of expensive but useful services.[86]

Combined effects of an aging population, medical technology, a vast number of new and effective drugs, social disorders, illegal drugs, and violence occurring concurrently in a brief period of time increased medical costs. At the same time,

---

[82] George H. Kraft. "In Defense of Health Care: Preserving the Capacity for Excellence." in *Beyond the Crisis: Preserving the Capacity for Excellence in Health Care and Medical Science* Henry M. Greenberg and Susan U. Raymond, editors. *Annals of the New York Academy of Sciences* 729, 1994, pp. 39-55.

[83] Cecil Pickett. "Impact of Health Care Reform on Research Innovativeness." in *Beyond the Crisis: Preserving the Capacity for Excellence in Health Care and Medical Science* Henry M. Greenberg and Susan U. Raymond, editors. *Annals of the New York Academy of Sciences* 729, 1994, pp. 106-110.

[84] Timothy Johnson. "Shattuck Lecture—Medicine and the Media." *New England Journal of Medicine* 339 (1998) 87-92.

[85] John Merline. "Pay or Pay: Managed care will not save Medicare, but a dose of reality might." *National Review* 29 May (1995) 45-48.

[86] William B. Schwartz and Daniel N. Mendelson. "Why Managed Care Cannot Contain Hospital Costs—Without Rationing." *Health Affairs* 11 Summer (1992) 100-107.

more and more could be done to relieve pain and suffering, prevention of disease, and delaying death in an era even more dramatic than that of the nineteenth century which produced one of the great epochs of medical advancement, along with unexpected social consequences of an aging and aged population. Better care and survival of disabled individuals made an enormous impact on families, including a spouse's ability to support both partners of a marriage with loss of financial support and health insurance.[87] Costs necessarily increased substantially.

---

[87] Peter T. Kilborn. "Disabled Spouses Increasingly Face a Life Alone and a Loss of Income." *New York Times* May 31, 1999.

Chapter VII

EARLY WARNINGS

VII. 1. EARLY SIGNS

In 1986, Maxicare Health Plan was rated best-managed health maintenance organization in the managed care industry. Within three years its founder resigned, filed for bankruptcy protection, and placed on *Financial World's* list of ten most poorly managed companies in the United States. With over two million enrollees in twenty-six states, bankruptcy of Maxicare dispelled the notion that only new, small managed care companies fail.

Managed care companies tended to underestimate incurred-but-not-reported (IBNR) claims or overestimate accounts receivable. As revenues fell behind outlays, the first response often was to draw on reserves from initial capitalization or through surpluses generated from operations. If no reserves existed or if exhausted, plans borrowed against credit assuming the shortfall to be temporary; at the same time, plans tried to improve short-run cash flow, delay or renegotiate contracts with providers to accept lower payment, tighten utilization review to deny care, drop unprofitable group contracts, bill employers earlier for premiums, or stall payments to providers. By changing accounting procedures used in its financial statements, a plan's deteriorating financial position could be concealed from regulators, investors, and contracting providers. Each of these tactics occurred abundantly in the managed care industry during 1980s and 1990s.

A managed care company's financial problems became known as result of complaints from providers about delayed payments for services rendered, when an excessive number of providers terminated managed care contracts, introduction of more stringent utilization procedures, or increased risk sharing—such as not returning the withhold to providers. At some point, financial condition of a managed care plan comes under scrutiny of state regulators who may take over management of the plan, require an external management team to "rehabilitate" the plan in an effort to maintain a viable delivery system and relationship with employers, search for a buyer, or liquidate the managed care plan.

Maxicare owed approximately $330 million to providers at the time of filing bankruptcy. State departments of regulation of managed care plans existed to protect enrollees, not to protect doctors or hospitals. First to be paid would be the state governments for costs of liquidation, then employees of the managed care company, followed by patients' claims, and last are other creditors including hospitals and doctors, if any funds are left. Since many states prevented providers from billing patients directly for services in case of managed care plan failure, physicians and other providers bore financial risk in event of managed care company insolvency. Laws of state versus federal jurisdiction in case of managed care plan insolvency is a complicated and unsettled issue.

Managed care plans may fail without becoming insolvent and still impose costs on involved parties, and failures tend to be underestimated. The number of managed care plans reached a peak of 679 between July 1987 and June 1988. Larger metropolitan areas were more likely to experience both managed care plan entries and failures. Greater numbers of managed care companies entering these communities produced intense price competition, which led to greater number of failures or mergers.

Although federal government regulates managed care industry through the Health Maintenance Organization Act of 1973 and its amendments, forty-two percent of managed care plans were not federally qualified in 1989. Amendments to Health Maintenance Organization Act weakened regulation, and budgetary limitations further reduced oversight of managed care plans. States, however, increased regulatory activity, especially the financial condition of managed care companies. In late 1980s, only 33 percent of HMOs were profitable, and 46 percent of well-established managed care plans were unprofitable. Increase in number of states that enacted laws and regulations following managed care plan failures parallels the pattern of failure and merger in the managed care industry.[1] All of this activity contributed nothing to providing services but added to overall cost of medical care.

In 1996, consumer surveys showed that the more mature a managed care market, the less satisfied consumers tended to be with managed care plans, such as claims handling, satisfaction with receiving care including referral to

---

[1] Jon B. Christianson, Douglas R. Wholey, and Susan M. Sanchez. "State Responses to HMO Failures." *Health Affairs* 10 Winter (1991) 78-92.

specialists. Those less satisfied were less likely to renew enrollment; any business with growing customer dissatisfaction risks defection of members.

In early managed care markets, utilization controls were less stringent than in mature markets. As markets matured, price competition between plans caused plans to be more concerned about limiting access and reducing costs leading to reduced access, referrals, and payments to physicians, which led to customer dissatisfaction. Even enrollees in mature markets who were satisfied with their plan were concerned about access to care and amount of time spent with their physicians. Allowing better access to physicians became a problem because it diluted the "brand" of a managed care plan.[2]

Many doctors and providers believed that expansion of managed care, investor-owned variety or non-profit, would have dire consequences, yet few spoke out. Instead, many accepted growth of managed care as a *fait accompli* and tried to position themselves and their institutions to survive. The managed care industry alienated physicians, undermined patients' trust of physicians' motives, hampered academic medical centers, handicapped biomedical research, and increased the number of patients without health care coverage.[3] Yet, managed care seemed an unstoppable force; several factors could limit its power: public demand of a greater choice of providers, a wave of anti-HMO sentiment in the press, backlash to gag-rules, "drive-through" deliveries, etc. A greater challenge to managed care industry's power lay in intensified competition, and growing strength of employer coalitions which put the managed care industry on the defensive. Unable to raise premiums, or forced to lower premiums, managed care plans became less profitable, reflected in lower stock prices, with a perception among investors that managed care companies were of doubtful value. Where managed care company profits were very low, plans merged to "achieve economies of scale," which is a failed concept.[4] The insurance industry was short-sighted by being hostile to physicians which was counterproductive in the long run, failing to understand that they were only as good as the product they sold, which was doctors, dentists, hospitals and other providers.[5]

The managed care industry responded to customer complaints by offering open access and alternative products for an added cost which may improve customer and physician satisfaction more than their policy statements, in which

---

[2] Louise Kertesz. "Trouble for HMOs?: Survey: Customer satisfaction falls as markets mature." *Modern Healthcare*. May 12 (1997) 48-51.
[3] Jerome Kassirer. "Managed Care and the Marketplace." *New England Journal of Medicine* 333 (1995) 50-52.
[4] Ken Terry. "You can thrive under managed care." *Medical Economics* April 7 (1997) 12-25.
[5] Mark Crane. "How low can fees go?" *Medical Economics* April 7 (1997) 26-47.

case where is the supposed advantage of 'managed care'? or 'managed cost?'—
patients still expect choice of physician and access to specialists. Once networks
of physicians, hospitals, and other providers were opened, managed care industry
could no longer justify its existence. The trend in health care insurance was a
return towards fee-for-service medical practice. Humana announced that it would
allow open access to every specialist in a particular city in the summer of 1997,
and abandon the gatekeeper altogether. Oxford Health named one of its open
access plans "Freedom Plan" and the other "Liberty Plan," diverting attention
away from deficiencies of managed care.[6] A managed care consultant said nothing
is wrong with paying doctors flat fees for medical care since there is no evidence
doctors will short-change care of patients. Thus, ethics and sense of responsibility
of doctors and hospitals kept managed care from being a greater disaster, not the
insurance industry.[7]

The greatest challenge to managed care plans came from incorporating risk
from Medicare and Medicaid populations, which Kaiser *Permanente* largely
evaded for decades. Government programs moved toward a managed care
approach to health care financing which placed pressure on managed care plans
geared to healthy populations. Crude control mechanisms such as pre-admission
screening and primary care gatekeepers proved ineffective and inappropriate for
chronically ill and high-risk persons who were increasingly enrolling in managed
care plans,[8] which raised the specter of rationing because rationing decisions must
be personalized since no two patients are alike and anticipated benefits of a given
treatment varies from patient to patient.[9] In 1998, two Medicare managed care
plans in Utah, one for-profit and one not-for-profit, failed with combined losses of
$24 million while covering only 20,500 enrollees giving a sobering warning to
other managed care companies.[10]

Some 'big players,' after much initial enthusiasm and bravado dropped out of
Medicaid managed care in some areas, including Aetna US Healthcare,
PacifiCare, Oxford Health Plans, Kaiser *Permanente*, Health Net, Tufts Health
Plan, Prudential, United Healthcare, Blue Cross and Blue Shield. Similarly, large

---

[6] Louise Kertesz. "Opening Access: HMOs' new tack leaves question, 'Where's the managed care?'"
   Modern Healthcare May 12 (1997) 40.
[7] Laura Mechler. "Higher co-payments keep HMO premiums down." *San Francisco Examiner* May
   4, 1997.
[8] Jeff Goldsmith. "A Different Health Care World Than Expected." *Health Affairs* 15 Winter 1996.
   109-110.
[9] A.S. Relman. "The Trouble with Rationing." *New England Journal of Medicine* 323 (1990) 911-
   913.
[10] Ron Shinkman. "Exit from Medicare: Intermountain, PacifiCare drop risk plans in Utah." *Modern
   Healthcare* June 22 (1998) 10.

managed care companies found Medicare managed care unprofitable with some notable exits by 'big players.'[11]

The managed care industry added to problems of voluntary and public hospitals by treating less than its fair share of indigent and uninsured patients[12]; managed care failed to improve community health. Like other managed care companies, Health Net spent nothing on medical research. It rejected a research project on ovarian cancer claiming that if it engaged in one aspect of research, other patient groups would demand research placing Health Net at a competitive disadvantage. Health Net's representative said that Health Net can't afford to pay for research if its competitors don't pay for research.[13] When hospital costs were relatively low, philanthropy and community contributions were a mainstay of support for public hospitals, but no longer.[14]

Managed care threatened to destroy many of San Francisco Bay Area's medical groups. In 1997, half of physician groups were bankrupt and the other half were dependent on subsidies from hospitals. Personal Choice Medical Group, one of the largest groups in the Silicon Valley, filed for bankruptcy protection in January 1997. Personal Choice signed up only 20,000 managed care enrollees but accumulated debt of nearly $3 million in a few years. At the same time, AHI Healthcare Systems, one of the Bay Area's largest IPAs in terms of doctors, was acquired by San Diego's FPA Medical Management, Inc., because it was close to financial collapse.[15] In July 1998, FPA, in turn, cascaded down declaring bankruptcy, followed by industry giant MedPartners. Meanwhile, managed care companies were subject to Wall Street's high profit expectations.[16]

In Minneapolis, three managed care plans dominated 80 percent of its managed care market causing business leaders and consumer advocates to question propriety of managed care companies since new health plans faced a few large competitors. Numerous conflicts of interest occurred when health plans owned hospitals and clinics which stifled competition. Cost reduction plateaued; overlapping allegiances made for a confused market, such that employers in the

[11] Peter T. Kilborn. "Largest H.M.O.s Cutting the Poor and the Elderly. *New York Times* July 6, 1998.
[12] A.S. Relman. "Meeting community needs is a major concern raised by for-profit health care." *Business and Health*. Jan/Feb (1985) 60.
[13] Erik Larson. "The Soul of an HMO." *Time* Jan. 22, 1996.
[14] A.S. Relman. "Shattuck Lecture—The Health Care Industry: Where is it Taking Us?" *New England Journal of Medicine* 325 (1991) 854-859.
[15] Chris Rauber. "Big squeeze puts doctors groups on critical list." *San Francisco Business Times.* Feb 7-13, 1997.
[16] Edward Martin. "Corporate medicine's huge losses produce doctor layoffs, chaos." *ACP-ASIM Observer* 18 (1998) 1, 18-19; Steven Heimoff. "After Shocks." *California Medicine* Feb/Mar (1999) 29-34, 62.

Twin Cities moved towards self-insurance.[17] Vertical integration of hospitals, physicians and health plans became the "grand illusion" in American health care.[18]

Cutting costs at any price failed in face of disintegrating quality of care, consumer dissatisfaction, physician revolt, and general exhaustion. Free-market mechanisms to control costs produced a vicious species of competition: "big, ugly buyers" grew to a size they were able to exploit providers. Employers and managed care plans won the upper hand, but not for long. Not all markets respond to pure capitation and competition. The market system of health care no longer underwrites or financially supports academic medicine, or the safety-net institutions of public hospitals. Managed care industry executives were rewarded by the market "for sticking it to hospitals and specialists" as they were expected to do.[19] Patients were cautioned not to confuse optimal medical care with what a managed care company claimed it would pay for—they were not the same.[20] Promoters of the managed care industry admitted that many patients, providers, and purchasers considered the health care system to be in turmoil, chaos.[21]

In April 1997, California Governor Pete Wilson appointed a task force to develop a comprehensive package of legislation to regulate managed care. Strangely, economist Alain Enthoven (a paid consultant to Kaiser *Permanente*) was appointed chairman whose concept of managed care favored marketplace competition. The result was a weak, feeble response. Over 100 bills had been introduced into the California legislature attempting to correct abuses of managed care.[22]

Well-documented favorable selection by managed care companies attracted younger, healthier members than fee-for-service plans. As managed care companies desperate for market-share signed up older and sicker populations, their costs and premiums rose sharply.[23] By taking increased risks, the managed care industry was in a bind to maximize profits leading it towards insolvency. According to a New York statute, directors of an insolvent insurance company are

[17] Jan Greene. "The Minneapolis Myth." *Hospitals & Health Networks* February 5 (1997) 56-60.
[18] J. Duncan Moore, Jr. "Expert spells doom for healthcare reform." *Modern Healthcare*. Mar. 18 (1996) 27.
[19] Moore.
[20] Carrie Sears Bell. "Dump Managed Care? This doctor did." *Medical Economics* April 28 (1997) 75-85.
[21] Paul M. Ellwood, Jr., and George D. Lundberg. "Managed Care: A Work in Progress." *Journal of the American Medical Association* 276 (1996) 1083-1086.
[22] Leigh Page. "Calif. task force could chart managed care's future." *American Medical News* Sep 15, 1997.
[23] Michael A. Hiltzik. "Are Executives at HMOs Paid Too Much Money?" *Los Angeles Times* Aug 30, 1995.

guilty of a crime; though extreme, the law reflects a broad policy of holding insurance company board members to an exceptionally high standard to avoid insolvency, and suits by regulators against directors of insolvent insurance companies are commonplace.[24] As more and more positions and offices mass movement into managed care were handed out, more and more inferior people occupied them so that hangers-on overwhelmed the movement, such as managed care utilization clerks and administrators, and mass movement's mission was dead.[25]

On brink of gaining full advantage, mass movements like managed care find themselves in dissension with violent life-and-death struggles against each other since the old enemy of fee-for-service medical practice was gone. Enmity became a habit; managed care companies made enemies of one another.[26] As breakdown approached, the managed care industry merged, competitors drove each other out of business, and borrowed and sold stock to the gullible.

VII. 2. EMERGING CRITICISM

A survey released in Feb. 1996, found that only 10% of consumers thought the managed care industry was "believable" which placed it last next to the tobacco industry.[27]

Claims of lower costs and improvement in care were banners of the managed care industry, however, in a study financed by managed care industry itself, evidence was mixed, such that both managed care proponents and opponents could find support for their positions on quality of care. On the other hand, evidence showed no pattern of worse quality of care. Health plans that developed a reputation for excellence in quality of care for difficult medical problems would attract new high-cost enrollees that brought with them only average premium payments which was a "recipe for bankruptcy," or at least a financially weakened company. Competitive pressures under fee-for-service could not be expected to result in cost containment, competitive pressures under capitation would not result

---

[24] John L. Akula. "Insolvency Risk In Health Carriers: Innovation, Competition, and Public Protection." *Health Affairs* 16 Jan/Feb (1997) 9-32.

[25] Eric Hoffer. *The True Believer: Thoughts on the Nature of Mass Movements.* New York: Harper & Row, 1951, p. 22.

[26] Hoffer. p. 133.

[27] Louise Kertesz. "HMO Makeover: Are managed care's efforts to overhaul its image too little, too late?" *Modern Healthcare* May 12 (1997) 36-46.

in improvement of quality of care.[28] Large employers were the critical party in health care whose contracts with managed care plans provided most citizens with health care coverage. Managed care plans competed on cost much more than on quality or any other professional standard, which tended to erode rather than promote quality.[29]

High medical bills did not make Hewlett-Packard less competitive any more than high food and housing prices in Japan make Toyota less competitive. Foreign exchange markets adjust value of dollars, yen and other currencies to neutralize effects of domestic costs: if costs of doing business in the United States rise, the dollar falls—and the United States will continue to export goods that it is relatively more efficient at producing. *Employees*, not employers, pay most of the cost of health insurance: employers' demand for labor depends on total cost of compensation, not the value of any one component. If benefit costs rise, wages will typically fall or rise less slowly to compensate. An understanding of these issues would not end the debate over health care financing but steer the debate to legitimate disputes.[30]

New circumstances alter demand for health care services. A marked increase in Medicare beneficiaries approaches as oldest baby boomers turn 65 in 2010. Technological developments presented new, expensive methods of prolonging human life. Six percent of Medicare patients who died each year accounted for 30 percent of Medicare costs. Among those who died, nearly 80 percent of costs occurred in the last six months of life. Since 1980s, providers continued cost shifting when Medicare first began economizing in earnest. As many workers covered by employer health-care plans know, the trend was toward fewer choices and higher contributions—largely the result of cost-shifting to the private sector forced by a combination of increasing demand for care from a growing elderly population combined with government efforts to reduce Medicare costs by paying less than actual costs, or a type of free-riding. A solution satisfactory to both was unlikely.[31]

With consolidation of HMOs, provider organizations found it harder and harder to achieve satisfactory agreements with ones that remained. In areas where only a few large managed care plans operated, nearly all doctors were in all plans

---

[28] Robert H. Miller and Harold S. Luft. "Does Managed Care Lead To Better Or Worse Quality Of Care?" *Health Affairs* 16 (1997) 7-25.
[29] Linda Emanuel. "Bringing Market Medicine to Professional Account." *Journal of the American Medical Association* 277 (1997) 1004-1005.
[30] Jonathan Marshall. "Health Care Economics Confuses Experts." *San Francisco Chronicle*. Jan. 15, 1996.
[31] Jerry Heaster. "Medicare dilemma is grim." *The Kansas City Star*. Sep. 29, 1995.

so that employers were unable to distinguish differences between plans.[32] Cost reduction achieved by most managed care plans had been modest at best and highly variable. In any case, no managed care plan was able to slow rate of increased costs.[33] Congress and Health Care Financing Administration (HCFA) have repeatedly said that they planned to reduce reimbursement to Medicare managed care plans by 5%. As more and more markets had only a few large managed care companies operating, most gains from intensified competition benefited stockholders and managers of managed care companies, not patients who sought treatment or health care professionals and personnel who provided medical services.

Rationing, or a restriction of services, was an unspoken method of the managed care industry. If a workable, medically sensible, ethically and politically acceptable rationing plan were devised, it would not save money in the long run. Each decision to restrict services temporarily reduces costs in one area of the system, but no single decision or group of decisions could halt increases in rest of the system that would cut ever more deeply into ethical medical practice. General opposition to further cuts would arise, and it would become apparent that rationing is not the solution to health care in the US. Managed care accomplished two of its goals: to restrict freedom of choice of specialists by enrollees, and to reduce the number of hospital admissions and length of stay, although decrease in hospital admissions is largely due to improved treatment and technology and not an effect of managed care. The emphasis on demanding shorter hospital stays produced minimal reduction of cost of hospital admission.[34]

The Welfare Reform Act of 1996 denied health insurance coverage to millions of poor people who previously had assured access to medical care through Medicaid. No reliable evidence suggested that Medicaid managed care would save significant amounts of money when providing coverage for the elderly, disabled, and chronically ill who accounted for about two thirds of all Medicaid costs.[35]

Physicians and hospitals faced a bewildering array of insurance plans that required large numbers of clerical personnel to handle massive volumes of

---

[32] Terry.

[33] A.S. Relman. "Controlling Costs by 'Managed Competition'—Would It Work? *New England Journal of Medicine* 328 (1993) 133-135.

[34] A.S. Relman. "The Trouble with Rationing." *New England Journal of Medicine* 323 (1990) 911-913; Paul A. Taheri, David A. Butz, Lazar J. Greenfield. "Length of Stay Has Minimal Impact on Cost of Hospital Admission." *Journal of the American College of Surgeons* 191 (2000) 123-130.

[35] Eli Ginzberg. "Managed Care and the Competitive Market in Health Care." *Journal of the American Medical Association* 277 (1997) 1812-1813.

paperwork. As hospitals and physicians adapted to a 'competition revolution' of 1980s, increased resources went to marketing, advertising, computer systems, management consulting, etc. which did not result in increased amounts of care.[36] If cautions were not taken by all parties, and should medicine's goal become maximizing shareholder returns, financial self-interest would not be a violation of ethical medical practice but would become the norm—a standard expected practice.[37]

Capitation by managed care was primarily a payment method—not a strategic direction. General Motors contracted with 115 managed care plans plus indemnity plans and PPOs. Its benefits manager said he was not concerned about capitation, but focused on overall quality and cost with a variety of payment methods, or a mix of methods; he was especially concerned about quality because providers were being asked to take on risk for things they cannot control, such as overall health of a population. A doctor with all healthy patients or all sick ones would result in either a windfall or a disaster for that doctor defying advocacy of 'managed competition' in which three, five, or more identical managed care companies vie with each other for market share.[38] Only 15 of 115 HMOs that GM offered achieved the automakers' 'benchmark' quality and cost status.[39]

A great deal of social distress lay ahead if business and government did not recognize adverse consequences of sociopathic, amoral economic forces of the managed care industry. Cross-subsidy financing of care provided to the uninsured would not be sustainable, and new public financing must be found to assist these populations and providers that serve them. Shifting more patients into the public hospital system was not a feasible option; many public hospitals faced deteriorating financial status, and their collapse would be hastened by movement of Medicaid into managed care.[40]

Senator Daniel Patrick Moyinhan (D-NY) warned that unless Congress acted to fund medical education and research through taxes on insurance premiums and transfers from Medicaid and Medicare trust funds, New York would no longer be

[36] V.R. Fuchs. "The Health Sector's Share of the Gross National Product." *Science* 247 (1990) 534-538.

[37] Gregg Easterbrook. "Healing the great divide: How come doctors and patients ended up on opposite sides?" *U.S. News and World Report* Oct. 13, 1997.

[38] Mark Crane. "What's holding back capitation?" *Medical Economics* Jan. 27, 1997.

[39] Susan Brink and Nancy Shute. "Managed care is pushing aside the private-practice doctors typified by TV's Marcus Welby or Dr. Kildare. What's replacing them isn't making anyone smile." *U.S. News and World Report* Oct. 13, 1997.

[40] Lynn Etheredge, Stanley B. Jones, and Lawrence Lewin. "What Is Driving Health System Change?" *Health Affairs* 15 Winter (1996) 93-104.

a center of medical innovation.[41] Academic medical centers developed a sophisticated, fragile structure of scientists, educators, and clinicians that conducted major research. Cost of care at these institutions was inevitably higher than at community hospitals because academic institutions trained health professionals, used the most sophisticated technology, treated patients with complicated illnesses, and subsidized research not funded otherwise. Fifty percent of the indigent received medical care at these institutions.[42]

Health Systems International, a managed care company, voiced the position of business through embracing managed care in a shift to "market-based system of focused, coordinated care." It expressed the position of business which wants to avoid care of the poor, medical education and research, claiming that investor-owned plans were spearheading change in the health care system with improved access, a strong emphasis on preventive care, affordability, and demonstrable quality—all disproved claims. A Health Systems International spokesman asserted that conversion of remaining nonprofit plans into investor-owned plans would provide funds for activities outside scope of the market.[43] Nevertheless, good medical practice requires extensive, unprofitable, even antiprofitable services, and that greed-is-good ethic of marketplace medicine forces the ill to be forsaken "imperiling the very soul of medicine."[44] Health Systems International argued that teaching medical centers were not entitled to larger payments because they have a pool of "cheap labor" in interns and resident physicians.[45] The managed care industry aimed to provide minimum health care cheaply as possible, however, they desired to avoid subsidizing teaching and research, or pay for expensive high-technology medicine that they would prefer their subscribers did not use. As funds from these sources disappeared, medical schools searched elsewhere for money to cover medical education and research.[46] National Institutes of Health, major research universities, tertiary medical centers, and private firms as well as private US industry supported astounding growth in

---

[41] Spyros Andreopoulos. "The Folly of Teaching-Hospital Mergers." *New England Journal of Medicine* 336 (1997) 61-64.

[42] Herbert Pardes. "The Significance of Health Care Reform for Research, innovations, and Academic Medicine." in *Beyond the Crisis: Preserving the Capacity for Excellence in Health Care and Medical Science* Henry M. Greenberg and Susan U. Raymond, editors. *Annals of the New York Academy of Sciences* 729, 1994, p. 134.

[43] Malik M. Hasan. "Let's End the Nonprofit Charade." *New England Journal of Medicine* 334 (1996) 1055-1057.

[44] David U. Himmelstein and Steffie Woolhandler. "Bound to Gag." *Archives of Internal Medicine* 157 (1997) 2033.

[45] Erik Larson. "The Soul of an HMO." *Time* Jan. 22, 1996.

[46] Spyros Andreopoulos. "The Folly of Teaching-Hospital Mergers." *New England Journal of Medicine* 336 (1997) 61-64.

biomedical research over the past generation.[47] The mass movement into managed care leaves one of the nation's great achievements—biomedical research—in a tenuous position when scientists and observers suggested that we have entered a new period of discovery and improvement in our ability to diagnose and treat the most complex medical problems.[48]

In 1997, the Department of Corporations (DOC) in California received an unprecedented $6.6 million augmentation to increase quality monitoring and oversight of California's managed care industry.[49] Between January and March 1997, the DOC fined 55 HMOs for failing to include the DOC's toll-free telephone line for patients' grievances. The large amount of managed care reform legislation reflected a lack of trust by patients and consumer of the managed care industry. Most consumers still trusted their doctors, but they don't trust insurance companies, and they don't trust HMOs. In years of rapid growth of managed care, health insurance coverage for children changed for the worse: in 1989, 26.4% of children were without private health insurance; by 1995, 33.9% of children were without private health insurance.[50]

Ballot initiatives in November 1996 failed to require managed care companies to prohibit such practices as gag-rules, financial incentives to providers to withhold services, insure safe and adequate staffing of hospitals, just cause for dropping providers, nurses and other caregivers, and in Oregon, to outlaw capitation altogether and to enforce 'any-willing-provider' initiatives. Some claimed the public was satisfied with managed care, though it may be more a matter of lack of public education than satisfaction with managed care. Campaign financing undoubtedly affected the outcome in that the managed care industry out-spent their opponents by 15 to 1. Referendum ballots usually require 4 to 5 years to develop enough public support to prevail on election day. The insurance industry runs a formidable number of advertisements whenever its business is threaten. To counter, opponents must not only have financial support to advertise, but also time needed to develop a broad movement in support of an initiative. The managed care industry claimed that the initiatives were not consumer-protection measures. In California, voters were asked to vote on two initiatives that had similar provisions, which probably split some of the vote. On the other hand, the California Medical Association sponsored two successful legislative initiatives:

[47] Rodney W. Nichols. "Research and Innovation: Introduction." in *Beyond the Crisis: Preserving the Capacity for Excellence in Health Care and Medical Science* Henry M. Greenberg and Susan U. Raymond, editors. *Annals of the New York Academy of Sciences* 729, 1994, pp. 95-105.
[48] Pardes. p. 135.
[49] *Physician Leader*. California Medical Association. No. 1623. Aug. 21, 1997.
[50] *American Medical News*. April 7, 1997.

banning physician gag-rules, and banning physician incentives for withholding care. Issues raised during the election were likely to become more lively, stimulated by reform movements and greater resistance on the part of the managed care industry.[51]

Federal and state governments seeking savings encouraged managed care by supporting enrollment of Medicare and Medicaid beneficiaries in managed care plans. At the same time, Congress, executive branch, state legislatures, media, and other parties were critical of the managed care industry. Strength of the resistance shook the managed care industry. In 1996, nearly 1000 bills attempting to regulate or weaken the managed care industry were introduced in state legislatures, and 56 measures were passed in 35 states. Federal administration became more aggressive in protecting those who enrolled in managed care plans under Medicare and Medicaid.[52] In 1997, more than one hundred laws were passed restricting managed care industry's clinical and legislative practices, such as Congress's mandated minimum 48-hour maternity stay, and dictated levels of mental health coverage, as well as outpatient mastectomies as another 'drive-through' procedure.

Legal Center for Patient Protection was formed which facilitates legal actions against managed care companies. Attorneys prepared class-action lawsuits charging fraud based on product warranty—that HMOs made promises they didn't deliver on, thus misrepresenting their product. Even within the managed care industry, that voluntary standards for the managed care industry were not sufficient was acknowledged; a national standard for managed care plans had been advocated.[53] Some physician groups, frustrated with tactics of managed care companies, began to unionize, saying that doctors should be caregivers and to help people through life's difficult times. Instead, doctors found themselves in a commercial model where patients produced a "revenue stream" for managed care companies.[54] Public trust was much more strongly invested in individual physicians than in the managed care industry.[55]

[51] Wayne J. Guglielmo. "Why the anti-HMO initiatives failed on Election Day." *Medical Economics* Dec. 9 (1996) 30-46.
[52] John K. Iglehart. "Health Issues, the President, and the 105th Congress." *New England Journal of Medicine* 336 (1997) 671-675.
[53] Louise Kertesz. "HMO Makeover: Are managed care's efforts to overhaul its image too little, too late?" *Modern Healthcare* May 12 (1997) 36-46.
[54] David Azevedo. "New owners drive this group to unionize." *Medical Economics* March 24, 1997) 194-196, 199-200, 205-207.
[55] David Mechanic. "Managed Care as a Target of Distrust." *Journal of the American Medical Association* 277 (1997) 1810-1811.

A serious threat to the managed care industry came from the possibility that employer purchasing groups would join together to negotiate directly with hospital and multi-specialty physician groups completely by-passing the managed care industry with repercussions of a significant decline of ability of managed care companies with their large debts to survive. The experience with direct contracting in Minnesota offered little promise because "care systems," as direct contracting is called, substituted one style of managed care for another. Experience with direct contracting was limited, but not encouraging.[56] The shift to managed care did not appear to be directly responsible for significant cost savings because, on average, managed care premiums were almost as high as those for fee-for-service plans.[57]

Changes in the health care system that resulted from the experiment of managed care are:

- Regulation of private practice of medicine by third-party payers.
- Interference with clinical practice decisions.
- Second-guessing and paperwork.
- Administrative delays in billing and collecting.
- Increased threat of liability litigation as a business relationship replaces trust and mutual confidence that characterized doctor-patient relationships.
- Threat of anti-trust violations.
- Advertising and slick marketing techniques encouraged by the Federal Trade Commission.[58]

A doctor writes, "...we need to remember the basics of the doctor-patient relationship and not fall prey to 'reformed' systems, which are fundamentally destroying that relationship."[59] Is managed care necessary? What level of complication is acceptable? How much harassment of public, patients and providers will be tolerated?

Most factors summoned to support claims of "crisis" in medical care have been present for years which blunts a "crisis" appellation because lack of

[56] Thomas Bodenheimer and Kip Sullivan. "How Large Employers Are Shaping the Health Care Marketplace." *New England Journal of Medicine* 338 (1998) 1084-1087.
[57] A.B. Krueger and H. Levy. *Accounting for the Slowdown in Employer Health Care Costs.* Cambridge, Mass: National Bureau of Economic Research Inc., 1997. Working Paper 5891.
[58] A.S. Relman. "Shattuck Lecture—The Health Care Industry: Where is it Taking Us?" *New England Journal of Medicine* 325 (1991) 854-859.

insurance portability, the barrier of pre-existing conditions, uninsured people relying on emergency rooms, and weight of medical insurance bureaucracy have been present for decades. One trigger for ruin of the managed care industry, other than political action, could occur with ending of the economic boom of 1980s and 1990s coupled with a wrenching nationwide "downsizing" of the work force exposing a large segment of the population to the deficiencies of the health care system: "The call to crisis finds a ready audience. But there are real dangers to crisis management. The urgent supplants the necessary; there are no horizons, only myopic visions."[60]

Highly excited mobilization of a mass movement like managed care is self-terminating: members grow weary; the host society reacts negatively and thwarts the movement's programs.[61] With gathering of experience, the managed care industry found it more difficult to hide its deficiencies, errors, and failed promise.

VII. 3. ROLE OF PATIENTS

The public was led to believe it could get something for nothing in managed care through a marketing strategy of little paper work and minimal co-payments. Denial must also be part of why the public joined managed care plans gambling that they would not need medical services. When illness occurred and when managed care members found that they may not get comprehensive treatment promised by managed care salesmen and saleswomen, they felt deceived and expressed their anger towards physicians and hospitals, when it was managed care managers and businesses who purchase managed care plans should bear their criticism. No wonder managed care salesmen and women were successful, up to a point, by promising services at a price that was unrealistically low while consumer magazines, business publications, general magazines, and newspapers endorsed the managed care industry.

After patients experienced restrictions imposed by managed care, they felt cheated. To cite W.C. Fields, you can't cheat an honest man, but easy if he has a

---

[59] William M. Bennett. "HMOs and Academic Medicine: Are They Both Deaf to Patients?" *Western Journal of Medicine* 166 (1997) 156.

[60] Henry M. Greenberg. "Three Threats to the Capacity for Excellence in Medicine." in *Beyond the Crisis: Preserving the Capacity for Excellence in Health Care and Medical Science* Henry M. Greenberg and Susan U. Raymond, editors. *Annals of the New York Academy of Sciences* 729, 1994. p. 9.

[61] John Lofland. Chapter 14 "White-Hot mobilization: Strategies of a Millenarian Movement." in James L. Wood and Maurice Jackson. *Social Movements: Development, Participation, and Dynamics*. Belmont, CA: Wadsworth, 1982. pp. 221-228.

touch of larceny in his heart. Patients came to expect more than the managed care industry could realistically deliver. In the process, patients became 'property' of managed care companies by being willing subjects, swayed by rhetoric of the managed care industry. Under managed care, doctors came to think of their patients as being "on loan" from managed care companies.[62]

Public dissatisfaction led to more consumer advocacy and activities in both public and private managed care plans. Growing numbers of elderly managed care enrollees alone increased pressure for consumer protection regulation. Managed care companies only recently became "mainstream" providers, and many treatment protocols, methods, and organizations were not suited to populations with greater medical needs. Consumer groups, particularly those working with disabled and chronically ill populations, realized that it was up to knowledgeable consumers and those working in their behalf to protect quality of services in managed care. Consumers tended to be more interested in knowing about physicians and hospitals than about managed care plans.[63]

Consumers behaved somewhat as a group placed in a bind just as physicians showing certain behaviors like any other group in a bind. Changes brought by mass movement into managed care did not deterred consumers from seeking medical care that might benefit them, nor did it stop development of technology to enable new interventions for patients' benefit. *Newsweek* reported that for patients, "HMO-style managed care unquestionably means limitations on the right—if it is a right—to request specific kinds of treatment." American patients and their families were quick to question their doctors, and quick to demand top-of-the-line care. Yet, the mass of consumers remained silent and submissive to the mass movement into managed care. Just as in other groups, apathy of masses was little more than a collective result of common, helpless submission to an outside, anonymous power of the managed care industry since few consumers have direct contact with a managed care company.[64] Consumer activism was generated by consumers' feeling that they could not trust their physicians to work solely in their best interest, combined with a mistrust of their employers and managed care plans.[65]

Yet, managed care was declared a mass movement, a 'revolution' in delivery of medical services and vanguard of the future by emotional rhetoric of managed care proponents. People transformed in presence of emotional arousal to follow

---

[62] Philip R. Alper. "Managed care, too, shall pass-the sooner the better." *Medical Economics* 17 June (1991) 93-96.

[63] Etheredge, Jones, and Lewin.

[64] "Doctore Under the Knife." *Newsweek* April 5, 1993.

[65] Etheredge, Jones, and Lewin.

advocates into managed care; and the more aroused they became, the more their thinking was non-analytical, concrete, and action oriented. Rhetoric during such excited states seems "obviously valid"; high confidence does not reflect accuracy or cogency of thought.[66] Although some economists and advocates of managed care claimed that insurance introduced the "perverse effect" of largely eliminating cost-consciousness by the public, consumers were fearful that the insurance industry, whether managed care or traditional, would in fact stand behind them in case of serious illness. Co-payments had relatively little restraining effect because serious illness runs up hospital bills well in excess of patients' expenses[67]—that is, after all, the purpose of insurance.

Under managed care, physician "paternalism," or long-term close relationships of patient and doctor, changed towards patient autonomy. As a result, some patients and their families claimed the right to aggressive, high-tech medical interventions which doctors might consider futile with little chance of achieving favorable results.[68] Others became "amateur physicians" with one case, themselves, creating more anxiety and terror than when the problem was entrusted to a personal physician.

Mass formations come into being and are held together by a common attraction, a leader or an idea, and by the tie created by common attraction of that leader or idea. Acceptance of leader or idea inflates self-confidence of adherents, making them immune to critical objections, particularly when the leader or idea procured step-by-step gratification of their urges. With any mass movement such as managed care, before enthusiasm slackens, the leader of the movement must call the mass together, and followers surrender themselves to a sense of omnipotence, are emotionally replenished, and envision themselves triumphant which is followed by a loosening of control, or a threat of returning to the old view. Objections make themselves felt, objections the individual, because of fear—of mass or leader—dared never express aloud, which instead had been overlaid by protestations of allegiance to the mass. Members of a mass are in perpetual alternation between surrender to blind emotions of the mass, and separation—even withdrawal—from that mass.[69]

[66] James E. Alcock. "The Propensity to Believe." in *The Flight From Science and Reason*. Paul R. Gross, Norman Levitt, & Martin W. Lewis, editors. *Annals of New York Academy of Science*. vol. 775. 1996. p. 67.
[67] John K. Iglehart. "From Research to Rationing: A Conversation with William B. Schwartz." *Health Affairs* 8 Fall (1989) 60-75.
[68] Lawrence J. Schneiderman, Nancy S. Jecker, and Albert R. Jonsen. "Medical Futility: Response to Critiques." *Annals of Internal Medicine* 125 (1996) 669-674.
[69] Sigmund Freud. *Group Psychology and the Analysis of the Ego*. 1921.

That the managed care industry pitted patients against physicians and physicians against managed care companies did not negate that patients benefit from cooperation among physicians and hospitals in both reduced costs and better service. Physician-patient relationship of trust is highly personal and intimate, similar in many ways to relationships within families, between teachers and pupils, or ministers and congregants. It is an "integrative relationship," one that depends on mutual recognition and acceptance of rights and responsibilities enforced by traditional norms as well as market pressures and government regulations. The "product function" of health is a peculiar one; it requires patients and health professionals to work cooperatively rather than as adversarial buyers and sellers. Adam Smith (1776) observed that mutual trust and confidence contribute greatly to efficiency of production. Thus, the model of "atomistic competition" as ideal in economics textbooks was not a proper goal for health care. Some refuted and decried a market solution to provision of medical care by the managed care industry, that the market alone could successfully seek out and establish both price and quality of care. In addition, dealing with death and dying exposes the problematic nature of standard, competitive solutions based on informed consumers and competitive suppliers.[70]

As the managed care mass movement, revolution, or mania spread, most consumers had little choice. Decisions on health plans were made by benefits managers of their employer's companies who were under pressure from company management and stockholders with little influence from employees. Many felt themselves trapped by the managed care industry with no options one way or another which led to the *Stockholm syndrome* when consumers faced no actual choice except between managed care companies, called "managed competition," i.e. competing managed care companies. Some companies centralized health plans into one managed care company, and changed annually according to price. Consumers could hardly be blamed when presented a one sided view by the managed care industry supported by a venal press. The public moved *en mass* into managed care willingly or unwillingly.

After more than four decades of a laudatory press, only in late 1990s was the public made aware of some of the most extreme examples of how managed care affected their medical care. Some employees put pressure on employers, but employees fearful for their jobs were not likely to protest vigorously, which may change if the economy remained strong with employees in demand and feeling more secure in their employment and opportunities for employment. The people

---

[70] Victor R. Fuchs. "The 'Competition Revolution' in Health Care." *Health Affairs* 7 Summer (1988) 5-24.

cheated in a mass movement are those expecting a new freedom, but freedom masses crave is not freedom of self-expression, but the freedom from intolerable burden of free choice and responsibility.[71]

Affluence increases interest in matters of health and medical care. In the eighteenth century, a physician said, "for those who have most comforts about them, are commonly the most comfortless of all mortals [for] those who want nothing else very commonly want health."[72]

---

[71] Hoffer. p. 129.

[72] Thomas Beddoes. *A Manual of Health: or, the Invalid Conducted Safely Through the Seasons.* London: J. Johnson, 1806. cited by Roy Porter. *Doctor of Society: Thomas Beddoes and the Sick Trade in Late-Enlightenment England* London and New York: Routledge, 1992, p. 62.

Chapter VIII

ACT FIVE

VIII. 1. LATE SIGNS

Traditional *prudential regulation* of health plans is based on the view that competition forces health insurance carriers to take too much risk. In managed care, health insurance carriers were criticized for taking too little risk and for competing in risk avoidance. Underwriting was restrained to healthy populations, and competition between managed care plans was encouraged. Regulators' and managers' of managed care plans concerns about insolvency risk dominated all other concerns because health care plans are subject to fiscal pressures common to all businesses in addition to insurance risks. Managed care plan insolvency did not recede as a policy concern because of complexities presented by managed care, which became more severe with pressures to reduce costs. As insolvency approached, efforts to keep managed care companies afloat shifted to protecting enrollees, or continuing coverage for which managed care plans could not pay.

Solvency is a governing business principle: an organization that does not bring in enough money to meet its obligations dissolves. Managed care company insolvencies generally are state proceedings, but because of ambiguity in the bankruptcy code, sometimes bankruptcies may be subject to federal bankruptcy jurisdiction.

The most common standard of solvency of an insurance company is *cash flow*—the availability of funds to meet obligations as they come due. The lag between collection of premiums and payment of related liabilities in health care insurance is about three months, whereas in other types of insurance the lag may be a number of years. Even a short period between collection and claims requires substantial reserves. A manage care company with $600 million a year in premiums must reserve approximately $150 million, i.e. thirteen weeks of premiums, in cash reserves to be solvent, called the 'prudential rule' of insurance. A managed care plan with $80 million in cash reserves, or six weeks of premiums, cash flow is satisfactory, but the managed care plan is "catastrophically insolvent." In 1982, the 'paradigm' of Kaiser *Permanente* reported cash reserves of 4 days, 9.6 days in 1992, and in 1998, its cash reserves were only 14 days; PHP managed care plan reported cash reserves as low as two days in 1998. The brief time interval of only three month lag in payments increased pressure for quick and accurate figures. Final settlement with private accounts takes a number of weeks. The expanding role of government as payer raised a new problem because with government payers final settlement is often years. Thus, decline in revenues may happen suddenly.

The tempo of change further threatened solvency of managed care plans since accounting based on experience provides poor guidance. In case of "incurred but not reported" (IBNR) losses, a managed care plan matches premiums and health care costs accrued to a closing date, but some providers' bills will not have been received by that date. Estimates of costs based on experience are usually wrong— IBNR is typically a large financial item. Different reasonable IBNR assumptions by managed care plans can double net worth or wipe it out. Rapid changes in health care financing due to movement towards managed care pushed the industry ahead of sound accounting principles that change more slowly. A managed care company with an aging Medicare population would be reflected in its financial statements, and an indemnity carrier would normally set aside a "loss reserve" which managed care plans routinely ignored.

Financial difficulty is a competitive disadvantage for any business, but financial problems are especially difficult for health insurance carriers, which become public record, except for privately held corporations like Kaiser *Permanente*. Purchasers of health care coverage feared effects of insolvency on continuity and quality of care. Providers were vulnerable because they continued to furnish care even when payment was in doubt. A distressed managed care company faced rapid deterioration of good will. Managers reporting to boards of directors and carriers reporting to regulators tended to understate bad news. Misappropriation is a rare but extreme threat to integrity, such as transferring funds into foreign bank accounts or living extravagantly on excessively high salaries and perquisites. Meanwhile, money could be used to hamper public oversight of managed care plans; generous campaign contributions and salaries for ex-regulators could sometimes buy a few years of relaxed scrutiny. Nor must insured persons suffer; current enrollee-claimants were treated generously since stealing from reserves could go on longer with an expanding subscriber base.

Money remained for a last, long run at better times, so long as no one noticed that reserves were disappearing or that debt was mounting. Nearly all managed care plans, including Kaiser *Permanente*, Oxford Health Plan, Health Net, Pacificare, and others, did not meet the prudential standard for financial solvency, whose reserves declined and debt increased.

With risk transferred to provider physicians and hospitals, providers were likely to be inexpert in managing this level of risk. Insolvency of doctors and hospitals was a serious public concern, especially inpatient facilities. A managed care company and providers sharing risk, dragging each other down, posed a double threat to continuity of care. Since risk-shifting could be used to avoid regulation, carriers were able to mask losses by transferring them to closely affiliated providers, but counter arguments seemed to have convinced most regulators. Development and interest in direct contracting, circumventing the managed care industry entirely, was largely a criticism of managed care plans.

Turnarounds of managed care companies in financial distress can achieve savings if utilization controls were lose and tighter methods were adopted, posing the hazard that a carrier in pursuit of a turnaround would under-fund care doing greater harm than if it closed down, especially since lose controls that could be further tightened were no longer possible. Generally, turnaround management of a business displayed a single-minded determination to cut costs with countervailing pressures in health care, especially ethical standards of providers and malpractice liability. However, excessive, irresponsible cost cutting did not require providers' complicity, and malpractice liability takes years to mature. Abuses became more likely with the move toward a system with less 'fat.'

Forbearance of health plans with no equity to lose could hope to survive only through high-gain/high-risk investments, gambling themselves further into debt while forcing more prudent health plans to take increased risks to match their premiums. Similar events would be expected of managed care plans in distress by taking greater and greater risks in an effort to forestall insolvency as seen in 1997 by the managed care industry when its investment in the long bull market doubled.

When a managed care plan deteriorates financially and runs out of funds to pay for care, focus shifts from keeping the plan afloat to protecting enrollees who face two problems: unavailability of care, and being billed for care that plans should have paid for. If providers render care expecting payment from a managed care company and payment is defaulted, providers usually have the right to bill patients, unless the plan obtained a *hold-harmless* agreement from providers that patients were not to be billed in case of collapse of carriers. Statutory hold harmless, which by law bars providers from recovering against insured persons, has been for the most part successfully opposed by providers who argued that they should not be a safety net for failures of the managed care industry over which they had no control.

Until recently, government's main concern in regulating managed care plans was protection of the public from insolvency risk, but the role of government became more complex. Cost, access, and competition emerged as more important issues. Government also became a purchaser of managed care services and a sponsor of health entitlements; thus, government programs may be weak in limiting short-term benefits in interest of long-term fiscal soundness.

In case of bank failures, with each wave of failures, dishonest bankers who were politically well connected came to light, which attracted publicity and political advantage. However, bank failures were not due to crooked bankers and politicians but to more fundamental institutional factors; and in the case of managed care, the multitude of errors and faulty basic fundamentals led toward insolvency. Avoiding blame was a powerful incentive for regulators which may be more important than doing a good job, i.e. ignoring a problem that would not surface until a successor was in office, or alleging private-sector malfeasance.

A consensus on role of providers in our health care system has not developed. Some view expertise and ethics of providers, physicians and hospitals, as a sound foundation for a health care system; others inclined to have more faith in government and regulation. For several decades, providers have been on the defensive, since antitrust laws restricted a collegial physician role in financing and delivery systems. Nevertheless, provider "fraud and abuse" was "criminalized" and blamed for health care costs.[1]

Congressional legislation to fund expansion and acceptance of health maintenance organizations in 1973 failed to achieve its goal of controlling costs. Although corporations moved steadily into managed care plans in 1980s, a deceleration of rising costs did not occur until the mid-1990s when managed care industry slowed its premium rate increases and retained 20 to 30 percent for "profit and expansion" previously discussed. Once enrollees were shifted to a less costly plan, savings were not duplicated, suggesting that further decreases must be accomplished by capitation of physicians, intensified use of preventive services, education of patients, and the use of clinical guidelines—each has been introduced and each has failed to reduce over-all costs. At beginning of 1997, the prevailing view became that health care premiums were likely to increase. Medicare planned to reduce payments to Medicare managed care plans by 7 percent, a correction for

---

[1] John L. Akula. "Insolvency Risk In Health Carriers: Innovation, Competition, and Public Protection." *Health Affairs* 16 Jan/Feb (1997) 9-32.

overpayment that resulted from managed care plan enrollment of a disproportionately healthy population. Medicaid costs would not be reduced by managed care.

Expansion of managed care depended on high profitability and ability to borrow capital. As profits decreased in face of competition with other managed care plans and the long stock market boom waned, ability to sustain capital needed for further growth of the managed care industry became doubtful, if not impossible. Experience alerted an increasing number of managed care enrollees, as well as the larger society, to risks that managed care mass movement represented to those enrolled. Public concern, discontent, and distrust grew as enrollees became aware of practices of the managed care industry. Rapid expansion into managed care did not prevent costs of health care from increasing by 5.4 percent in 1995 to double-digit increases in 1998. In the fifteen years from 1980 to 1995, a time when managed care grew rapidly, overall health care costs quadrupled from $250 billion to $1 trillion in current dollars.[2]

Managed care emerged as discounted insurance based on agreements between managed care companies and providers, however, discounts that slowed inflation substantially reduced providers' capacity to deliver uncompensated care that was essential to access and stability in providing health care coverage. Providers delivering care to the uninsured served as a safety valve for both health care delivery and the political system, enabling the nation to avoid social confrontation due to conspicuous, widespread suffering resulting from unavailability of medical care. Uncompensated care was reduced by as much as 36 percent in areas with a high penetration of managed care and reductions in public funding. Reduction of uncompensated care occurred because discounted prices that providers were forced to give the managed care industry eliminated financial margins that providers once received from private payers to cover uninsured patients. Private insurance premiums historically represented cost of care for insured beneficiaries plus a little more for care of others. Consolidation of the market under managed care enabled private insurers to refuse this cost shift, which was advocated by some economists and spokespersons for the managed care industry. Although the amount of uncompensated care declined, need increased.

Decline in private insurance was particularly disturbing given the healthy economic context in which it occurred. Insurance was discontinued in the public sector as well, increasing pressure on providers, such as changes brought by welfare reform and care of legal immigrants. Cuts in Medicare and Medicaid

---

[2] Eli Ginzberg and Miriam Ostow. "Managed Care—A Look Back and a Look Ahead." *New England Journal of Medicine* 336 (1997) 1018-1020.

further reduced indirect subsidies for uncompensated care. Discounts to managed care companies put health care providers under unprecedented pressure to maintain services; reduction in services seemed inevitable leading to adverse social effects. Providers would not be able to sustain discounts demanded by the managed care industry, resulting in a return of increases in medical costs. Increased direct costs to Americans by out-of-pocket payments, higher co-payments, deductibles, etc. combined with growth of the uninsured population indicated that market solutions were not solving but masking underlying problems of structure and financing in the health care system to produce both savings and expansions of coverage. With the shortcomings of the marketplace, the US was on brink of a major collision between increased need and reduced capacity of providers to deliver health care services resulting in financial instability in the health care system. The marketplace system of managed care reduced ability to provide uncompensated care but created no mechanism for providing it.[3]

As the "paradigm" of managed care failed, managed care proponents tended to disregard negative data, and claimed that stories were ignored of millions who were "disenfranchised," and emphasized claims that the managed care industry "dramatically" increased prenatal education, lowered infant mortality rates, elevated percentages of children's immunizations, took the lead in annual mammograms, detected undiscovered illnesses, and established quality measurement, and health care consistency "heretofore unmatched,"[4] which mistakes compliance for quality, and repeats unsupported, exaggerated claims as pointed out earlier. Since managed care created little incentive to treat patients, managed care plans pursued "cost-effective care." Money saved by reducing "unnecessary surgery, excessive inpatient days, preventable illnesses, and so on can be directed toward better prevention, and care,"[5] all disproved claims.

An ominous possibility became creation of a managed care company that was too big to be allowed to fail. Such events occur in banking in that large banks cannot be allowed to fail because it would disrupt the entire economic system. New York State provided a cash infusion to Empire Blue Cross in 1993 which may have played a role in keeping the managed care industry alive for a longer time.[6] With large increases in premium rates by Kaiser *Permanente*—up to a 12

[3] Barbara Markham Smith. "Trends in Health Care Coverage and Financing and Their Implications for Policy." *New England Journal of Medicine* 337 (1997) 1000-1003.
[4] Ross K. Goldberg. "Afflicting HMOs: Why do media ignore managed care's achievements to focus on horror stories?" *Modern Healthcare* May 12 (1997) 34.
[5] Robert Kuttner. "Must Good HMOs Go Bad?" *New England Journal of Medicine* 338 (1998) 1558-1563, 1635-1639.
[6] V.R. Fuchs. "Managed Care and Merger Mania." *Journal of the American Medical Association* 277 (1997) 920-921.

percent or higher increase in annual premiums charged to its customers since 1998 to make up loses, screened fundamental problems,[7] it nears the point where Kaiser *Permanente* and other managed care plans can't be allowed to fail and must be bailed out with a massive infusion of money since no HMO-of-last-resort is available, except by the printing of more paper by another managed care company. Business was likely to expend more money in a vain effort to "save the appearances" of the failed managed care "revolution."

Apposite to the managed care mass movement are manias in financial institutions; crises are bound up with transactions that overstep the confines of law and morality, shadowy though those confines may be. The propensity to swindle and be swindled run parallel to a propensity to speculate during a boom: "Crash and panic, with their motto *sauve qui peut* [stampede, panic], induce still more to cheat in order to save themselves"; the revelation of a swindle, theft, embezzlement, or fraud often signals panic.[8] Enough of each occurred in progression of the managed care mass movement to draw attention of public, profession, and government but were over-looked, disregarded, and ignored leading towards a crisis, a crash: "Crisis does not necessarily purge a system of folly; old habits and attitudes die hard."[9]

VIII. 2. RE-CAPITULATION

Just when bizarre, confounding, irrational conditions brought by managed care seemed to be overwhelmingly bewildering, frustrating and infuriating, the managed care mass movement began to make sense. The history of managed medical care followed a familiar pattern:

- Managed care was promoted to doctors as a way to make money, at least to remain in practice, and to business as a way to increase profits by appealing to greed.
- Those caught in managed care enthusiasm recruited others to join.
- A revolution declared that swept away resistance, obstructed critical evaluation.
- Supportive data turned up.

[7] Carl T. Hall. "Kaiser Raises Key Group's Rate 10.75%." *San Francisco Chronicle* June 12, 1998.
[8] Charles P. Kindleberger. *Manias, Panics, and Crashes: A History of Financial Crises.* Third Edition. New York, Chichester, Brisbane, Toronto, Singapore: John Wiley, 1996. p. 66.
[9] Barbara W. Tuchman. *The March of Folly: From Troy to Vietnam.* New York: Ballatine, 1984. p. 208.

- Contrary data ignored or discredited.
- Cautions neglected.
- Regulatory agencies and silence of the courts supported a managed care mass movement.
- Managed care fed on itself as an "unassailable truth" to become its own version of the truth.
- Those in managed care plans—patients, providers, and purchasers—thought they could beat the odds, or get out in time if anything went wrong.
- Enthusiasm for managed care expanded beyond its capacity to stretch and accommodate bogus, discredited data based on a tower of logical errors.
- Unattended by new awareness by public, providers, and government, managed care like other mass movements hastened to its ultimate conclusion.

Enthusiasm for and contagion of the managed care mass movement followed a familiar pattern of irrational human behavior seen many times.

As presented here, the 'health maintenance organization' was a conceptual and practical failure: the case against traditional medicine was exaggerated and never established, the case for managed care was contrived and declared against evidence and experience, recurring financial failure of managed care companies, failure of competition to provide medical services, 'appearance' of quality satisfied proponents of managed care, fallacy of efficiency, fallacy of prevention, decline of financial resources, longer delays to pay claims, credit withdrawn, the bubble bursts with many hurt—both patients and providers, the new "paradigm" of managed care fails:

> A scientific paradigm may remain dominant throughout a protracted crisis during which bothersome anomalies continue to accumulate. But another way of making the same point would be to say that paradigms do crumble when their unfruitfulness has become overwhelmingly evident.[10]

Managed care's outstanding feature was its *lack* of innovation. Old values and standards of medical practice were declared "suddenly invalid" with a cynical attitude towards illness, patients, and profession. If thesis presented here is correct, providers who "embraced" managed care risked accumulating accounts

---

[10] Frederick Crews. "Freudian Suspicion Versus Suspicion of Freud." Greenberg. "Humanities" in *The Flight From Science and Reason.* Paul R. Gross, Norman Levitt, & Martin W. Lewis, editors. *Annals of New York Academy of Science.* vol. 775. 1996, p. 472.

receivable from managed care companies that will never be paid, threatening their survival and leaving many patients without physicians and other medical services. The "greater fool theory" of managed care applies in that managed care companies must pay off maturing claims with new money. Kaiser *Permanente's* CEO David Lawrence's statement that "Kaiser must grow" is more appropriate than he might have thought; without growth in young and healthy or healthy Medicare population, it faced decline.

I conclude that the rush into managed care, the so-called evolution that became a so-called revolution, an irrational, value-oriented mass movement resulted in a grotesque, sociopathic, failed social experiment.

A similar phenomenon paralleling developments in medicine occurred in an anti-intellectual movement in science education. All but most elementary rudiments of science, mathematics, and engineering have been removed from curricula of most college students which is "traceable in large part to negligent acquiescence by scholars, intellectuals, teachers, administrators, and above all, by the scientists themselves."[11] Thus, learned helplessness and passivity are not exclusive behavior of physicians; the striking "stony silence" of the science and technology community, similar to *Fallacy of the Quietest, or No Complaint*—if no one complains, no one suffers, or the error of *supinity*[12] that allowed rise of a muddleheaded managed care mass movement to gain wide acceptance.

Non-medical people may not appreciate how little could be done for patients before the 1930s. Development of sulfanilamide and antibiotics in the 1930s was the forefront of technological revolution in health care.[13] Conditions changed drastically during five decades of development of managed care. Medical costs will never go back to days of six percent of the Gross Domestic Product—unless the Gross Domestic Product doubles.

The community of science and medicine might be more easily swayed by a powerful demagogue than by a less charismatic person with a more powerful truth; when such circumstances occur, they are part of the reason:

> ...why some paradigms materialize in the first place and part of the reason
> why some survive for what we all see as a remarkably and embarrassingly

---

[11] Gerald Holton. "Science Education and the Sense of Self." in *The Flight From Science and Reason*. Paul R. Gross, Norman Levitt, & Martin W. Lewis, editors. *Annals of New York Academy of Science*. vol. 775. 1996, p. 552.

[12] Neal F. Lane. quoted by Holton. p. 551.

[13] George H. Kraft. "In Defense of Health Care: Preserving the Capacity for Excellence." in *Beyond the Crisis: Preserving the Capacity for Excellence in Health Care and Medical Science* Henry M. Greenberg and Susan U. Raymond, editors. *Annals of the New York Academy of Sciences* 729, 1994, pp. 39-55.

long period of time in retrospect. We also embrace [!] shared beliefs out of our own various needs, and we wonder later how we ever came to think that 'X' was 'Y'.[14]

In case of failures of financial institutions, a lender of last resort, *dernier ressort*, must be ready to halt a run out of financial assets into money by making more money available to halt the run on assets.[15] No such last resort exists in medical care.

Our profession placed in a bind reacted with passivity, supinity, and defensiveness lacking conviction of our ancestral colleagues, rather than believing in ourselves and the work we do, for Avicenna (tenth century A.D.) said, "...it is painful for them to see my merits beside their ignorance." Learned helplessness and risk-averse behaviors do not and cannot serve either our profession or our responsibility to patients and public.

At what point might the irrational mass movement into managed care have been averted or contained? Once critical and realistic evaluation of Kaiser *Permanente* ceased in 1948, the groundwork was set for development of an irrational mass movement. The approval given to managed care's unreason by the prestigious *New England Journal of Medicine* and other publications added to momentum towards and suppression of critical appraisal of managed care. A realistic assessment prior to the Health Maintenance Act of 1973 might have altered the course of events, but the HMO Act institutionalized error. Physicians did not comprehend the seriousness of the threat and did little; what protest occurred became distorted by the press into self-serving criticism by doctors, which perversely became a sanction of the managed care industry, and led to medicine's ultimate surrender into "preferred provider" lists by physicians in 1982.

Medicine's failure to respond cannot be attributed solely to doctors or medical societies, but like academic institutions and the science community, physicians failed to educate the public on the nature of what was in store for them by mass movement into managed care. Once in full bloom, the mass movement of managed care, like other mass movements, could not be altered by argument, reason or appeals to common sense. Rapid conversion into managed care, its failing financial status combined with extraordinary rapid growth, set the stage for a crash.

---

[14] Bruce M. Psaty and Thomas S. Inui. "The Place of Human Values in the Language of Science: Kuhn, Saussure, and Structuralism. *Theoretical Medicine* 12 (1991) 345-358.

[15] Kindleberger. p. 146.

The mass movement into managed care was somewhat more complicated than other mass movements due to interaction of numerous masses with overlapping and conflicting interests, goals and subconscious motives: masses consisting of doctors, dentists, hospitals, other providers, managed care companies, medical group practices, individual and small associated medical practices, elected government officials, government bureaus, business interests, investors, each group of payers, and patients. The individual acts consciously, the mass—into managed care—acts unconsciously. Critical intelligence along with lack of conviction and passion are the main obstacles to action by the mass, which were over-come by suggestion and mass propaganda that necessarily makes use of language that is allegorical and full of images of simple, straight-forward, imperative, and certain formulas focused on a vague, idealized future that never materializes.[16]

VIII. 3. HISTORICAL PARALLELS

We can add managed care to an extensive, frightful list of irrational mass movements, the legions of examples of crowd psychology, such as the Mississippi scheme of John Law, the South Sea company in England, tulipomania in Holland, gladiola mania in Holland, the fern craze in England, gold fever in America, nineteenth century medical quackery, twentieth century medical quackery, Florida land boom of 1910, Ponzi's postal scheme in 1920, Home Stake Mining in 1964, a similar scheme in Ohio in 1985, junk bonds, the bubble economy in Japan in the 1990s—each with a superficially logical structure based on false premises, the list is endless with common features: the schemes are similar with no innovative features. Such schemes were defined by Hyman Minsky "as a type of financial activity engaged in when interest charges of a business unit exceed cash flows from operations."[17]

Managed care demonstrated characteristics of a classic scheme: enthusiasm, gullibility, avarice, recruitment, contagion, traditional methods invalidated, protective agencies subvert, courts silent, warnings ignored, feeds on itself, frenzy, can't fail, must grow or collapse. The entity of managed care, as proposed here, became a irrational mass movement, an extraordinary popular delusion that

---

[16] Serge Moscovici. *The aged of the crowd: A historical treatise on mass psychology.* Translated by J.C. Whitehouse. Cambridge, London, and New York: Cambridge University Press, 1985, pp. 90-91.

[17] Kindleberger. p. 66.

became a madness of the crowd.[18] The appearance of one—such as Kaiser *Permanente*—produced others of a similar kind, such as Health Net and Aetna US Healthcare.

While John Law's plan was at its height of popularity, people "wise in their own conceit," crowded in thousands to ruin themselves with frantic eagerness by the famous plan for paying off the national debt with paper money.[19] The firm of Overend, Gurney in England, which crashed on Black Friday in May 1866, was said to consist of "sapient nincompoops."[20] Bubbles may or may not be swindles. John Law was not a swindler, but based his theory on two fallacies: that stocks and bonds were money, and that issuing more money as demand increased was not inflationary[21]; the same principle as a failing managed care company selling more paper in the form of stock to raise capital to forestall collapse.

A parallel development to the managed care mass movement occurred in the research science environment in academia[22] and the growth of postmodernism which rejected the principle of reason of the Enlightenment, and denied possibility of objective knowledge.[23] Over the past three decades, universities were infiltrated by enemies of learning, intellectual rigor, and empirical evidence who "pass off political opinion as science and engage in bogus scholarship." Managed care, similarly, must be considered anti-intellectual, anti-medicine, and sociopathic.

Members of a mass movement do not act in accordance with their conscience or show their best side—often showing the opposite. Instead of individuals coming together and improving, their good qualities tend to diminish and deteriorate, falling towards that of its lowest members, which means that all are equals. The mass acquires not qualities of the 'average,' but qualities of the 'lowest common denominator' measured by standards of those who have the least and obey the lowest instincts.[24]

[18] Charles Mackay. *Memoirs of Extraordinary Popular Delusions and the Madness of Crowds.* 1841 and 1852. Reprint. Foreword by Bernard Baruch. New York: Farrar, Straus, and Giroux, 1932, p. 88.
[19] Mackay. p. 49.
[20] Kindleberger. p. 22.
[21] Kindleberger. p. 71.
[22] Henry Greenberg. "Introductory Remarks." *The Flight From Science and Reason.* Paul R. Gross, Norman Levitt, & Martin W. Lewis, editors. *Annals of New York Academy of Science.* vol. 775. 1996, p. x.
[23] Paul Kurtz. "Two Sources of Unreason in Democratic Society: The Paranormal and Religion." in *The Flight From Science and Reason.* Paul R. Gross, Norman Levitt, & Martin W. Lewis, editors. *Annals of New York Academy of Science.* vol. 775. 1996, p. 494.
[24] Moscovici. p. 14.

VIII. 4. PRECIPITATING EVENT

A precipitating event that would signal fall of the managed care industry cannot be known, but a number of possibilities are here considered:

- A rise of insurance company ethics.
- Government regulation.
- Legal remedies.
- Breakdown of ERISA protections.
- Competition from other types of insurance.
- Direct contracting.
- Wall Street will turn its attention elsewhere.
- Medical society protest or a physician's union.
- Doctor rebellion.
- Burnout of medical personnel.
- Decline in quality.
- Outrage.
- Patient revolt.
- Social unrest. Rebellion of the masses.

The precipitating event could be a combination of several or all of those listed above which is not a complete list of possibilities. If the managed care mass movement follows the course of other manias and mass movements, no precipitating event need occur. A mass of people rapidly join a mass movement such as managed care, but come to their senses slowly and one at a time, so that a gradual withdrawal of support weakens the movement until it cannot sustain itself. A sudden, massive withdrawal is not likely, according to the historical nature of popular delusions and irrational mass movements, but a gradual, sustained decline brings about collapse. Le Bon says, "Behind the constant mobility of the crowd, behind its furors, enthusiasms, violences and hatred generating so much upheaval, there persist very tenacious conservative instincts....This double tendency–revolutonary in actions, conservative in feelings–is generally overlooked by their leaders."[25]

---

[25] Gustave Le Bon. *Les Opinions et les Croyances*. Paris: E. Flammarion, 1911, *Opinions and Beliefs*. in *Gustave Le Bon: The Man and His Works*. Editor Alice Widener. Indianapolis: Liberty Press, 1979, pp. 199-200.

Failure of the delusion of the managed care mass movement may have a cleansing effect that, if taken correctly, allows for healing and renewal, belatedly and at a high price.

VIII. 5. COLLAPSE OF THE BUBBLE

Managed care failed conceptually, intellectually, financially, politically, popularly, and in medical practice. The "miracle of capitation" proved to be a sham marvel, a miracle of rhetoric and deception. Managed care was regressive since it looked back to 1940s and 1950s when medical care was simpler, expectations lower, and accomplishments modest. In 1980s and 1990s, masses of people moved into managed care plans while the managed care industry, for-profit and not-for-profit, struggled against insolvency. The "intellectual underpinnings" of managed care contained so many logical errors and disproved claims as to be meaningless, a muddleheadedness that was destructive to rational planning, belonging in the same category with cold fusion, spoon bending, deconstruction, and magical thinking. We can expect advocates of managed care to behave like those who have advocated similar delusions who are faced with reality: the quack, lashed back at his physician-tormentors claiming "Persecution!"

Attention to criticisms of arrogance, greed, and excessive paternalism restrained doctors from defending the profession's strengths. A venal press focused on fraud though rare, and the less rare scrupulously suspect physicians who over-charged Medicare and other insurance plans. The pervasive inability to distinguish profession from practitioner inhibited defense of professionalism.[26] As criticism of managed care mounted, the managed care industry formed the Health Care Information Institute, an inflated title for managed care industry's propaganda, which objected to the sentiment that the fee-for-service era was a "golden age" and they needed to "kill this notion" by the error of *Imputation of Bad Design* to undermine existing norms and institutions, asserting that without managed care "employers would no longer provide coverage," an *argumentum ad metus* or appeal to fear.[27]

When failures of mass movements occurred, promoters disappeared. Some were persecuted by mobs. Some fled their native countries. Some died in poverty and disgrace. Flight was one form of exit, suicide another. A number of managed

---

[26] Greenberg. p. x.
[27] Ron Shinkman. "Defending managed care: Coalition works to reverse health plans' negative image." *Modern Healthcare*. October 26 (1998) 38.

care executives have fled from the US after failure of their schemes, and at least one exited by suicide. The tragic figures in history of mass movements are zealots and promoters who lived long enough to see downfall of the old order by actions of the mass.[28]

Managed care's essential character was its disregard for and violation of the rights of others, with fear, deceit and manipulation as central features. We cannot expect advocates and promoters of managed care to accept responsibility for consequences of their actions, but to show a callous lack of empathy, grandiosity, a lack of remorse without a sense of guilt. With glibness and superficial charm, using a facile jargon, they are more likely to direct blame elsewhere,[29] to blame victims themselves for being foolish or deserving their misfortune, and to minimize harmful consequences of their own conduct; or they may be indifferent, callous, cynical, and contemptuous towards rights and suffering of others.[30]

Proponents of managed care, perhaps at beginning, may have believed that they were on a crusade. The business community and some in government were ready disciples and jumped on the bandwagon. In this respect, "The charlatan resembled his dupes; his, too, was a weak and disappointed nature that sought consolation in the realm of illusion, on a plane that was no longer that of the sober earth."[31] Some university scholars, expert and famous in academic specialties, readily "embraced" peddlers of managed care; business executives and claims managers whose planning horizons seldom project beyond three months saw an opportunity for further profits. Headlong plunge into folly of managed care by business was led Allied Signal, by 'embracing' managed care in 1987; Allied Signal was followed by the herd instinct of business executives, often in highly charged emotional tirades against their benefits managers, without concern for long-range implications.[32]

Physicians, in some instances, and public, too, succumbed to the rhetoric of managed care promoters: "For naturally the best men are the least suspicious of fraudulent purposes."[33] By a betrayal of public trust and confidence, promoters of

---

[28] Eric Hoffer. *The True Believer: Thoughts on the Nature of Mass Movements.* New York: Harper & Row, 1951, p. 129.

[29] Carl B. Gancono and J. Reid Meloy. *The Rorchach Assessment of Aggressive and Psychopathic Personalities.* Hillsdale, New Jersey and Hove, England: Lawrence Erlbaum Assoc, 1994, p. 3.

[30] *Diagnostic and Statistical Manual of Mental Disorders.* Washington, DC: American Psychiatric Association, 1994, pp. 645-650.

[31] Grete de Francesco. *The Power of the Charlatan.* New Haven: Yale University Press, 1939. pp. 27-28. in James Harvey Young. *American Health Quackery.* Princeton, New Jersey: Princeton University Press, 1992, p. 4.

[32] George Anders. *Health Against Wealth: HMOs and the Breakdown of Medical Trust.* Boston and New York: Houghtn Mifflin, 1996, pp. 16-34.

[33] Thomas Hobbes. *Leviathan* Indianapolis: Bobbs-Merrill, 1958, p. 20.

the managed care mass movement deliberately induced confidence in its adherents toward an improbable, glorious future:

> Worse still, the [Nixon] administration's [HMO] plan was an open door to charlatans and get-rich-quick artists. The monthly prepaid premiums of many thousand subscribers add up to a handsome sum of money, and the prospect of establishing a skeletal plan, quickly building a large enrollment, collecting the prepaid premiums, and then either prolonging the plan's life and profits by skimping on service or collapsing the plan and skipping town with the cash was bound to attract the unscrupulous....some entrepreneurs were quite content to make a killing and then disappear.[34]

People yield to such propaganda during times of stress, pain or sorrow. In absence of exact knowledge or insurmountable difficulties, a credulous person craves a miracle, and is ready and willing to be overwhelmed by the personality and claims of managed care promoters. The promoters may be as self-deluded about their powers as victims, but eventually become aware of failures while continuing to promote the delusion of the movement, consciously deluding those who trust and depend on them. Aided by those previously duped, the credulous are reluctant to acknowledge the fact and magnify promoters' apparent successes. Pain or fear of pain, as well as vanity, are particularly vulnerable to opportunities of unproven remedies and crackpot solutions.[35]

For promoters of the managed care industry, mass movement into managed care afforded a new "get rich scheme" by claiming to offer "something for nothing" or, at least, an unrealistic claim to provide comprehensive medical services when such was not intended. Gullibility and a high standard of living make for easy and lucrative marks. Others, exploiting cupidity of the public, advocated managed care with false pretenses in the same category—each bilks profits from the gullible by gaining confidence, and building a logically structured argument on a base of false data and fallacious assumptions.

A mass movement retains its vigor if it offers nothing to the present, but to posterity. When invaded by those who want to make the most of the present, the 'mission' of the movement is dead. The movement must concern itself with the frustrated, to reconcile them to the present, to make them meek and patient, offering a distant hope and vision: an instrument of power and opiate for the frustrated.[36] If wisdom were operative, re-examination and re-thinking, a change

---

[34] Lawrence D. Brown. *Politics and Health Care Organization: HMOs as Federal Policy.* Washington, DC: The Brookings Institution, 1983, p. 421.
[35] *Encyclopædia. Britannica.* (1971) 9:819.
[36] Hoffer. p. 138.

of course was possible; however, when failure begins to appear in a mass movement, initial principles rigidify, which leads to increased investment and need to protect egos. Policy founded upon error multiplies—it does not retreat. The greater the investment and the more involved the sponsors' egos, the more unacceptable is change and disengagement. Pursuit of failure enlarges damages, or the "wooden-headedness of those headed for tragedy."[37] In mass movements such as managed care, Dr. Le Bon cautioned:

> Every general belief being little else than a fiction, it can only survive on the condition that it be not subjected to examination. Even when a belief is severely shaken, the institutions to which it gave rise retain their strength and disappear but slowly. Finally, when the belief lost its force, all that rested upon it is soon involved in ruin.[38]

"God's interference" does not acquit man of folly; rather, it is a device for transferring responsibility for man's folly. In the absence of a god, the managed care industry, like other businesses, projected its folly to claims about shortcomings of computer systems and managing data. The collapse of managed care, though it bring tragedy and suffering, should not be feared, but expected, for it is a sign of progress, however painful.

VIII. 6. CURRENT CULTURAL TRENDS

When reason sleeps, the monsters of human pride, foolishness, malice, and cruelty emerge to do their worst.[39]

Unreason that plagues academia, concurrent with the mass movement of managed care, is a product of the delusion of and craze for "radical postmodern theory" in the humanities, which is blamed as a source of discontent with reasoned inquiry, called "faddish nihilism"[40]; such muddleheadedness, or "post-

---

[37] Barbara W. Tuchman. *The March of Folly: From Troy to Vietnam.* New York: Ballatine, 1984, p. 383.

[38] Gustave Le Bon. *Psychologie des Foules.* Paris: F. Alcan, 1895, *The Crowd: A Study of the Popular Mind.* Atlanta: Cherokee Publishing Co., 1982. p. 143.

[39] Paul R. Gross and Norman Levitt. *Higher Superstition: The Academic Left and Its Quarrels with Science.* Baltimore and London: Johns Hopkins University Press, 1994, p. 215.

[40] Henry Greenberg. "Humanities" in *The Flight From Science and Reason.* Paul R. Gross, Norman Levitt, & Martin W. Lewis, editors. *Annals of New York Academy of Science.* vol. 775. 1996. p. 443; Alan Sokal and Jean Bricmont. *Fashionable Nonsense: Postmodern Intellectuals' Abuse of Science.* New York: Picador, 1998, p. 183.

modern anti-intellectualism" in decried by academicians as "orthodoxy of intellectual complaisance."[41] Anthropologist Margaret Mead cautioned that the United States was entering "a new Dark Ages of medieval mysticism and mumbo-jumbo, of belief based on self-interest, mob politics, and fear rather than research and open-minded inquiry," which is congruous with the managed care mass movement: "A brand of anti-intellectualism is running amok..."[42] which is amply shown in writings of some economists and other managed care advocates. A mathematician was more sardonic in conditions within the world of academia: "Windbags, bluffers, and moral one-uppers are having a field day. The daft and the silly are raised on high."[43] Timidity and ineffectiveness of scientists and scientific societies to counter attacks against them condemned the feebleness of their attempts to understand the attacks, and to oppose them.[44]

The re-engineered corporation, another example of a mass movement that infiltrated the business community on baseless claims, seldom, if ever, increased market share, increased profits, or decreased expenses—all the supposed purposes of re-engineering, yet businesses re-engineered at the cost of hundreds of millions of dollars largely because their competitors re-engineered, and gained fortunes for top management. Charlatanism in business advice exists for the same reason it did in pre-scientific medicine: people are desperate to be told there are easy answers to complex business questions that they "suspend their skepticism" still dominated by a "preponderance of non-sense."[45]

The managed care mass movement and assault on reason by the managed care industry and its spokespersons can be seen in context of larger, more pernicious movements within society and business community, especially academia to which the nation should look for guidance and pursuit of rigorous investigation that tenure and academic freedom afford. When academic institutions give way to unreason, phenomena like managed care expand without critical appraisal or restraint.

The managed care mass movement fits well in the history of folly; the perennial nature of folly is apt to thesis presented here. One can't help but react in conflicting ways: that the managed care industry was sociopathic with its sanction of illusion, and astonishment that so many were so readily deceived and corrupted.

---

[41] Christopher Ricks. *Essays in Appreciation*. Oxford: Oxford University Press, 1996, p. 294.
[42] William A. Henry, III. *In Defense of Elitism*. New York, London, Toronto: Doubleday, 1994, p. 3.
[43] Norman Levitt. "Mathematics as the Stepchild of Contemporary Culture." in *The Flight From Science and Reason*. Paul R. Gross, Norman Levitt, & Martin W. Lewis, editors. *Annals of New York Academy of Science*. vol. 775. 1996, p. 48.
[44] Holton. p. 552.
[45] Graham Topping. "New Model Business." *Oxford Today* 10 (1998) 11-13.

Mass movements do not pursue truth: they demand illusions, and cannot do without them, giving what is unreal precedence over what is real, influenced by what is untrue as much as by what is true, tending not to distinguish between the two.[46] Hardly anyone made a greater blunder into folly than earnest Dr. Relman at *New England Journal of Medicine* in 1993, saying, "I particularly applaud ['managed competition'] recognition that insurance subsidized by employers or government must inevitably be capitated and delivered by organized groups of physicians."[47] Allied Signal blundered enthusiastically, without restraint. In June 2000, the Supreme Court of the United States found in favor of the managed care industry and its policy of "rationing" because managed care has been promoted by Congress since 1973. When failure begins to appear, initial principals rigidify, leading to increased investment: the pursuit of failure enlarges damages.[48]

The movement into managed care could not be stopped. Whole populations converted into managed care with little protest acting like a single mass. Once deceived by managed care advocates, providers as well as patients claimed that they were tricked or swindled. Each mass movement follows Schiller's dictum, which states: "Any one taken as an individual, is tolerably sensible and reasonable—as a member of a crowd, he at once becomes a blockhead."[49] Yet, out of folly and breakdown of the irrational mass movement of managed care can come valuable experience: "But it is through the malice of this earthly air, that only by being guilty of Folly does mortal man in many cases arrive at the perception of Sense."[50]

---

[46] Sigmund Freud. *Group Psychology and the Analysis of the Ego.* 1921.
[47] A.S. Relman. "Controlling Costs by 'Managed Competition'—Would It Work?" *New England Journal of Medicine* 328 (1993) 133-135.
[48] Sarah A. Klein. "Justices validate HMO pay incentives." *American Medical News.* June 26, 2000; Tuchman. p. 383; M. Gregg Bloche and Peter D. Jacobson. "The Supreme Court and Bedside Rationing." *Journal of the American Medical Association.* 284 (2000) 2776-2779.
[49] Mackay. p. 48.
[50] Herman Melville. *Pierre: or the Ambiguities.* (1852). New York: E.P. Dutton, 1929, p. 233.

Chapter IX

AFTER THE FALL

IX. 1. CARRYING ON

What came of the managed care misadventure? We learned that patients could be moved from physician to physician and from managed care plan to managed care plan somewhat reluctantly, but with little protest; that the public can be fooled but not forever. The medical care "product" of today bears little resemblance to medical care a half-century ago at beginning of the managed care industry. Millions of hospital days were saved by outpatient surgery unrelated to managed care; outpatient surgery did not have its impetus from managed care: better anesthesia, better medicines, better pre-operative evaluations lessened risks of outpatient surgery.

"Managed competition," i.e. competing managed care plans, encouraged medical care management by insurance companies. However, cost-effective care was best provided by competent and compassionate physicians with no incentive to do more or less than appropriate, which requires training, experience and judgement. To be cost effective, responsibility was best placed in hands of doctors and their patients.[1] Professional medical care means assumption of responsibility for patients' welfare, a physician who values patients' welfare above his or her own despite physical discomfort or inconvenience.[2]

---

[1] A.S. Relman. "Controlling Costs by 'Managed Competition'—Would It Work?" *New England Journal of Medicine* 328 (1993) 133-135.

[2] John H. McArthur and Francis D. Moore. "The Two Cultures and the Health Care Revolution: Commerce and Professionalism." *Journal of the American Medical Association* 277 (1997) 985-989.

Fear and divisiveness were the *modus operandi* of the managed care industry during a period in history of medicine that was bizarre, senseless, an eclipse of common sense. While some doctors followed managed care zealots and men-of-words, many did not. Many individuals in mass movements standby without becoming involved with the movement, and remain in the movement out of inertia even though they had defected in spirit, waiting for an opportunity to withdraw with minimum conflict and publicity.[3] What was innovative about managed care that could justify claims that managed care was a "revolution" and that "managed care is here to stay"? Nothing. The only sense to be made of claims by proponents of managed care is its lack of sense—a strange chapter in the history of medicine, but an ordinary occurrence in the history of human folly, a miracle of rhetoric, and ascendance of knavery.

Only an unreformed optimist could believe that the marketplace would restrain and contain medical care costs in face of aging of US population, medical complexity and remarkable technological interventions.[4] Most economic markets are healthy, but some suffer "economic pathology"; believers in market rationality contended that a market corrects its own mistakes and that it was better at learning than government. But markets failed to learn many lessons over past three centuries, which makes one doubt whether markets learn lessons from the past; occasionally, rarely, governments learn.[5] One has a persistent feeling that enough resources are available in this country to do what physicians and medicine are called upon to do if done reasonably by all concerned.

After fall of managed care, will public and profession be on guard against turning medical care over to the same knaves who assaulted propriety with managed care? Or resume referring to physicians as physicians instead of 'providers,' patients as patients instead of 'capitated lives,' patients' needs as patients' needs not 'plan costs,' and medical care as medical care instead of 'consumption of health care resources'? The more successful prevention becomes the greater over-all costs by extending life, which entails *increased* medical costs. Fundamental questions remain: what will consumers and employers choose to reward? How will available services be organized? Who will determine clinical

[3] Gardner Lindzey and Elliot Aronson. *The Handbook of Social Psychology.* 2nd ed. Vol. 4. Reading, Mass, Menlo Park, CA London, Amsterdam, Don Mills, Ontario, Sydney: Addison-Wesley, 1968, p. 595.

[4] Eli Ginzberg. "Managed Care and the Competitive Market in Health Care." *Journal of the American Medical Association* 277 (1997) 1812-1813.

[5] Charles P. Kindleberger. *Manias, Panics, and Crashes: A History of Financial Crises.* Third Edition. New York, Chichester, Brisbane, Toronto, Singapore: John Wiley, 1996. pp. 201-202.

practices? And on what basis will it compete?[6] Regular indemnity medical insurance plans received no support or sanction, but showed a modest comeback in spite of massive promotion of managed care.

In a commercial market, less affluent populations do without expensive goods; in medical care, no such population exists—need is universal.[7] Scientists and doctors will have to ally with intelligent non-scientists and non-physicians, and "learn how to turn aside the rhetoric of the Luddites, uncongenial as that task may seem."[8] Those who advocated managed care have their mortality, too, and medicine is a small world. We all have the courage to endure someone else's illness, and to say that someone else consumed too many medical resources.

As early as 1978, it was said that increase in health spending was due to growth in public and private insurance coverage with access of many who previously did not have insurance, including the aged and the poor, as a result of advances of technology in prolonging life and enhance quality of life. New coverage was provided, e.g. mental health, alcohol and drug abuse, health-care workers' pay was brought up to levels of other industries; that "the growth in spending should not mislead one into thinking it is all bad."[9] That is, costs that are not in the control of physicians and cannot be compassionately controlled by government or managed care except by refusal of services on basis of costs.

Can ruin be averted? Possibly, but the natural history of delusions and manias of irrational mass movements leads to tragedy, destruction, and ruin. Those physicians and hospitals with large and growing accounts receivable from managed care companies risked survival.

I have outlined my thesis on chaotic conditions in provision of medical services in the US. The backing and filling, finger pointing, backbiting amongst managed care advocates will not be pleasant to witness. Those who think costs should not enter into decisions about medical care will be disappointed. A return to reasonable fee-for-service alone will not change a growing demand for medical care by an aging population for whom we can offer more and more effective therapies, which confronts an unwillingness to pay costs. The Post-Managed Care Era promises to be equally challenging.

---

[6] Lynn Etheredge, Stanley B. Jones, and Lawrence Lewin. "What Is Driving Health System Change?" *Health Affairs* 15 (1996) Winter 93-104.
[7] McArthur and Moore.
[8] Barry R. Gross. "Flights of Fancy: Science, Reason, and Common Sense." in *The Flight From Science and Reason.* Paul R. Gross, Norman Levitt, & Martin W. Lewis, editors. *Annals of New York Academy of Science.* vol. 775. 1996. p. 80.
[9] A.C. Enthoven. "Consumer Choice Health Plan." *New England Journal of Medicine* 298 (1978) 650-658, 709-720.

IX. 2. CONTINUING PROBLEMS

A change in US industrial productivity occurred in the early 1990s, with 'downsizing' of the labor force in many large corporations, reducing levels of middle management and personnel wherever possible. Bottom lines of companies were enhanced without aiding problems of the economy as a whole, in particular worsening income distribution as well-paying jobs declined as entry-level jobs rose. The country experienced many other problems—the deficit, a weakening infrastructure with deferred maintenance, a slowdown in innovation except in high technology and finance with cutting corners and mismanagement in the latter which Kindleberger says may indicate that United States is in the process of losing its world economic position.[10] Health care professionals were expected to provide services for persons with emotional disorders, marital strife, addictions, and other problems that previously were in the province of families or religious communities.[11]

If the trend in aging continues, by 2010 only 0.8 persons will pay into Medicare for each person covered.[12] Aging of post-World War II baby boomers and persistence of relatively low fertility levels will further reduce ratio of workers to Medicare beneficiaries, along with longer life expectancy. While young and middle aged people generally require episodic care, frail elderly suffer multiple chronic diseases, functional disability, and nursing and psychosocial problems that require complex multidisciplinary care, and respite care for caregivers.[13] At beginning of the twentieth century, ten children (under age eighteen) lived in the US for each person age 65 or older; by 1960, the ratio was four to one; and by 1990, two to one, and the ratio continues to fall.[14] Nursing home costs account for almost 1% of the Gross Domestic Product illustrating how social trends affect consumption of medical services.[15] Aging is a product of favorable sociopolitical conditions and a stable economy along with prevention,

---

[10] Kindleberger. p. 188.
[11] V.R. Fuchs. "The Health Sector's Share of the Gross National Product." *Science* 247 (1990) 534-538.
[12] James E. Orlikoff. "Future Trends in Health Care: How Will They Affect Rheumatologists?" *Highlights* American College of Rheumatology October 18-22, 1996. p. 16.
[13] Howard Fillit. "Geriatrics and Health Care Reform: Opportunities in Managed Care for Preserving Excellence in the Care of the Elderly." in *Beyond the Crisis: Preserving the Capacity for Excellence in Health Care and Medical Science* Henry M. Greenberg and Susan U. Raymond, editors. *Annals of the New York Academy of Sciences* 729, 1994. p. 178.
[14] V.R. Fuchs. "The Clinton Plan: A Researcher Examines Reform." 13 *Health Affairs* Spring (1994) 102-114.
[15] Fuchs. (1990).

successful medical interventions, effective drugs, and sophisticated technology, which add to concerns for providing health care to the frail elderly.

Most elderly die of progressive chronic illnesses in advanced old age after a long period of disability. Care of the dying involves medical evaluation, advanced planning, life-extending treatments, satisfaction of patient and family, quality of life, family burden, survival time, provider continuity and skill, and bereavement support. That all of us will die, all have an interest in being confident that our suffering and pain will be compassionately cared for, and that we will find our time at the end of life part of the experience of being loved and finding meaning. Care of terminally ill individuals accounts for 10 percent of costs of health care. Managed care incentives turned end-of-life issues upside down with growing fear that doctors were being paid *not* to do things, and a danger of getting too little care at a time when patients were in greatest suffering and least able to fend for themselves. No matter which way courts rule money issues will continue to hover about end-of-life medical care under managed care.[16]

End-of-life decisions risk being directed by health plans, government regulation, and institutional policies. In case of futile care, treatment may be deemed inappropriate. At what level of assurance can the chances for success of treatment be arbitrarily set by third parties without consent of patients or patients' doctors? Futile care redirects the entire relationship because health plans, government, or other payers may not pay for it.[17]

Hippocrates said that the art of medicine consists of relieving sufferings of the sick, lessening violence of their diseases, and refraining from attempts at cure when patients were overmastered by disease. In 1505, Francis Bacon urged physicians to treat patients' symptoms not only when they might recover, "but also when, all hope of recovery gone, it serves only to make a fair and early passage from life."[18] Care of the terminally ill, primarily the elderly, is not a problem physicians alone can solve, but the matter must be decided by society.[19] To restore balance between physicians' obligation to prolong life and obligation to relieve suffering, we must acknowledge a peaceful death as a legitimate goal of medical care and an integral part of a physician's responsibilities. A Supreme Court opinion requires that laws do not obstruct provision of adequate palliative

---

[16] Gloria Shur Bilchik. "Dollars & Death: Money changes everything. Now it's entering the debate over the right to die—with explosive results." *Hospitals & Health Networks* Dec. 20, 1996.

[17] Mark Siegler. "Falling Off the Pedestal: What Is Happening to the Traditional Doctor-Patient Relationship?" *Mayo Clinic Proceedings* 68 (1993) 461-467.

[18] Daniel P. Sulmasy and Janne Lynn. "End-of-Life Care." *Journal of the American Medical Association* 277 (1997) 1854-1855.

[19] Diane E. Meire, R. Sen Morrison, and Christine K. Cassel. "Improving Palliative Care." *Annals of Internal Medicine* 127 (1997) 225-230.

care, especially alleviation of pain and other physical symptoms of people facing death.[20] Nevertheless, a managed care company spokesman objected to end-of-life care saying that it was not a payment dispute, but a "philosophical dispute about how much pain and misery you should be able to inflict on a patient who is terminally ill."[21] Ethics of the marketplace, practices of managed care, conflicted with the assertion of John Ruskin (1862): "THERE IS NO WEALTH BUT LIFE. Life, including all its powers of love, of joy, and of admiration."[22]

Trust of physicians entails dealing with criticism and defending ourselves, rights of patients, and the profession. The original causes of delusion of the managed care mass movement remain; cost increases were claimed to be due to irresponsibility of physicians and patients while ignoring actual causes of increased costs. However, legislative activities about managed care showed that managed care's period of uncritical sanction in Washington was over because of concerns about quality of care rendered under managed care, and doubts over long-term cost savings, although Federal agencies maintained a commitment to managed care.[23] The task was more daunting when regulatory officials and courts were part of the mass movement of managed care.

The market as normally understood is not allowed to function in health care, but it does not mean that market forces have no effect. Special expertise of those who provide health care makes them difficult to regulate and typically want more resources than society wants to provide. Control of such systems is difficult because rarely does a bureaucrat know enough about work providers do, and when they do, rarely can they measure work they do understand, and when they do have measures, they may be over-whelmed with data. Almost everybody believes money could be saved by eliminating "waste," but one person's waste is another person's vital service, and administrative cost controls of undisputed waste may exceed savings. Societies have not solved these problems with police, firefighters, generals, or college professors, so expectations in managing doctors and hospital administrators should be modest. No reform will work in terms posed by both health care and budget reformers: a 'rational and efficient' allocation of resources although a changed attitude reflected a genuine resistance toward managed care. Increased legislation and regulation of managed care deepened and

---

[20] Robert A. Burt. "The Supreme Court Speaks: Not Assisted Suicide but a Constitutional Right to Palliative Care." *New England Journal of Medicine* 337 (1997) 1234-1236.

[21] Michael A. Hiltzik and David Olmos. "Do HMOs Ration Their Health Care?" *Los Angeles Times*. August 27, 1995.

[22] John Ruskin. "Ad valorum." from *Unto This Last*. (1862) London and New York: Penguin Classics, 1985, p. 222.

[23] Peter P. Budetti. "Health Reform for the 21st Century? It May Have to Wait Until the 21st Century." *Journal of the American Medical Association* 277 (1997) 193-198.

perpetuated the muddleheaded movement in a desperate effort to save appearances of a failed social experiment.[24]

IX. 3. THE ROLE OF BUSINESS AND INDUSTRY

Pacific Business Group on Health began in 1989; it emphasized access to care, treatment outcomes, patient satisfaction, administrative process, and appropriateness of care.[25] Measures advocated by the Group on quality did not measure quality, but measured compliance. Members of the Group said that business had no commitment to managed care and that they were aware of abuses in management of managed care, but maintained their allegiance to managed care industry because short term price was considered "cheaper," and were satisfied to choose between managed care companies solely on basis of price.

Society's approval of managed care that relieved business of "pass-through costs" conflicting with altruistic ideals of medicine and financial imperatives of business would eventually resolve in favor of business by corporate personnel whose jobs and future depend on maintaining corporate profits.[26] Mutually dependent, medicine and business coexisted through the ages in a "necessary tension." The marriage of business and medicine is not optional, but, for better or worse, necessary.[27] Medicine cannot be practiced in a financial vacuum.

If business and industry succeed in averting medical expenditures for research, education, and pass-through costs by means of managed care, a new source of funding must be found. If public hospitals fail due to lack of funding, social and political consequences could be grave, such that socio-economic conditions in the United States may decline with drastic effects on business and industry. If all funding for care, research and education were to fall to federal, state and local governments, higher taxes would erase any conceived or alleged savings claimed for the mass movement of managed care.

Since causes behind increased medical costs were misrepresented by advocates of managed care, pressuring providers into submission proved an unsatisfactory and costly remedy, and mis-directed the debate by overlooking behavior of mass movements. Medical care remains care of the ill and injured;

---

[24] Budetti.

[25] *1996 Report on PBGH Quality Initiatives.*

[26] A.S. Relman. "Practicing Medicine in the New Business Climate." *New England Journal of Medicine* 316 (1987) 1150-1151.

[27] Linda Emanuel. "Bringing Market Medicine to Professional Account." *Journal of the American Medical Association* 277 (1997) 1004-1005.

what is reasonable and ethical does not change according to payment sources whether fee-for-service, managed care, or public assistance. The actual causes of cost increases to be dealt with openly and honestly:

1. *Business desires a lesser burden in costs for the elderly, including retirees.*
   Business is caught in a bind in that success of the business and economic state allowed better living conditions that improved health and increased longevity with attendant rise in over-all health care costs. In early twentieth century, retirees died soon after retirement, but not today—some companies have as many retirees as employees.

2. *Care of the poor under Medicaid is especially onerous to business and industry because they are neither employed, nor do they contribute to the tax base but draw from it*
   Medicaid was the first payment program to be underfunded. It has been kept alive by the provider community who assumed much of costs of the Medicaid program. Increased funding for hospitals under Medicaid occurred in late 1970s when many inner-city hospitals were threatened with closure. No similar increase in funding occurred for physicians by Medicaid. Business carried a minimal share of this cost. Unless at least break-even payments are provided, the Medicaid program is threatened.

3. *Care of the uninsured is also born by physicians and to some extent by other insurance payers.*
   An overcharge is necessary to cover costs of the uninsured; few uninsured individuals are able or willing to pay for either office care or emergency care. Business carries little direct obligation for these costs and avoided these extra costs by means of managed care.

4. *Managed care proceeded under the assumption that if Medicaid and Medicare could get away with under-funding, then managed care industry could also get away with under-funding, why should business pick up the additional tab?*

5. *A reduction in unnecessary and wasteful administrative costs would be welcome to business whether in health care or their regular business activities.*
   Administrative costs of managed care plans were enormous. In addition, each hospital had multiple layers of administrators, case managers, utilization review personnel, and attendant support personnel and costs that do not produce services to patients. In addition, each doctor's office

under managed care required increased number of personnel to deal with managed care plans.

6. *End of life care was born principally by Medicare and Medicaid, not directly by business.*

   Often labor intensive, emotionally draining on families and medical personell, care cannot be put into a production line. Although the 'down-slope of the curve,' terminal care by physicians, nurses and other medical personnel can be gratifying and uplifting by being medical attendants at death of a courageous or heroic patient that can't be measured in production dollars.

7. *Care of families of workers has long been a benefit of many corporations and industries in recruiting and retaining valued employees.*

   Since most family members are relatively young, and most are healthy, costs to employers were not unreasonable. Productive capacities of employees can be enhanced indirectly by providing medical care for family members.

Effective solutions to the problem of increased health care costs must take into account:

- False premises of managed care, and failed "intellectual underpinnings."
- Excessive costs of administration.
- Pass-through costs from Medicaid, Medicare, uninsured, and under-insured.
- Technological advances that are effective in medical care, sometimes astonishingly so.
- An aged and aging population with multiple, complex disorders and co-morbidity.
- Greater complexity in therapies.

By succumbing to seductive rhetoric and persuasiveness of advocates of managed care, business and industry allowed the managed care industry to gain its sanction based on false and failed claims. The public expected what should be taken for granted: reasonable care at a reasonable price—not restrictive, regressive, wasteful tactics of the managed care industry.

In 1998, premium charges by managed care plans to businesses reached "double digit inflation" with increases of ten to fifteen percent or as high as 22 percent, "employers faced a health-care market in turmoil."[28] Transferring responsibility for purchase of health insurance from employer to employee would provide for genuine freedom of choice, although tax-exempt status of health insurance would be a difficult but not insurmountable obstacle.

IX. 4. COMING TO OUR SENSES

Many physicians view any constraint on resources a violation of their professional trust. Making physicians allocate some resources does not reduce their professionalism, but relies on it. Trusting physicians may seem risky, but even when responding to financial incentives, physicians strive to provide adequate care.[29] Professionalism, as earlier noted, remains the best method of surveillance of physician offenders. Two percent or so of physicians would abuse any system; they are readily identified and tend to be recidivists. Yet, controlling errant practitioners is as difficult in medicine as in any other group or profession in a liberal society. Controls designed to free ethical practitioners could not develop under managed care, which assumed all physicians were errant and irresponsible: the error of *argument ad invidiam* or *The Opposer-General's Justification.*

Matthew Arnold (1862), citing Bishop Thomas Wilson, says "Firstly, never go against the best light you have" or initial interest in the concept of managed care; "secondly, take care that your light be not darkness."[30] After a half-century of the mass movement of managed care, we see that light of the managed care mass movement was, in fact, darkness. That quackery, poverty, bigotry, and violence remain primary and stubborn challenges to our intelligence and will, is applied equally to managed care: "Realizing that progress may not happen, that unreason plays a crucial role in many impulses to act, our confrontations will not be easy. But at least we will be looking at our problems in a more realistically sophisticated way."[31]

We cannot expect either government or business to abandon managed care, nor doctors or insurance industry to object strenuously. However, the best hope is

[28] Joseph B. White and Rhonda L. Rundle. "Big Companies Fight Health-Plan Rates: Employers Demand HMOs and Hospitals Cut Costs." *Wall Street Journal* May 19, 1998.

[29] Joseph White. "Markets, Budgets, and Health Care Cost Control." *Health Affairs* 12 Fall (1993) 44-57.

[30] Matthew Arnold. "Doing As One Likes." from *Culture and Anarchy.* ed. J. Dover Wilson. Cambridge University Press, 1932, p. 96.

[31] James Harvey Young. *American Health Quackery.* Princeton, New Jersey: Princeton University Press, 1992, p. 31.

in the people, an informed public, as occurred in California in 1975 with the professional liability ('malpractice') insurance crisis that threatened to curtail availability of medical care in their communities. An informed, involved public faced with losing medical services, acting through the representative process, has potential to be an effective body in opposition to the managed care mass movement. An informed public will act, and government and medical insurance industry will be forced to listen,[32] despite intimidation by the managed care industry.

How much do we pay for health? Nearly all commentators agreed that 12 percent of the Gross Domestic Product going to medical care was "unsustainable." Since nearly all aspects of society relate to health, including education, housing, defense, law enforcement, transportation, agriculture, clothing, and recreation our "bill for health" is closer to 99.9 percent of the Gross Domestic Product. In an affluent, civilized society, how much of our resources should reasonably be devoted to medical care remains problematic. Revelations of waste, fraud, duplication, abuse, inefficiency, and profiteering by the managed care industry can be stopped, but only by the will of an informed and active public.

To have practiced medicine during the time of madness of a crowd was a daunting experience when it seemed that all were swept away by a one-sided argument, by muddleheadedness, by woodenheaded embracing of the mass movement of managed care. Yet, muddleheadedness is the sovereign force in human affairs, more potent than malevolence or nobility. Muddleheadedness blunts wisdom, misdirects compassion, clouds insight, and is the chief artisan of unintended consequences of human history: "To crusade against muddleheadedness, therefore, may be the most futile, and hence the most muddleheaded, quest of all....Still, passivity in the end is more reprehensible than quixotry."[33] Science and medicine lapsed into silence and supinity, but stirrings of resistance and alternatives began to be heard.

According to the nature of mass movements, an organized counter-mass movement against managed care is not likely to develop, or if organized, has little chance to succeed. Following behavior of irrational, value-oriented mass movements, individuals of a mass slowly come to their senses, out of an "hypnotic dream" while under the illusions of the primitive, collective subconscious of the primal horde in the mass movement of managed care.

---

[32] The staff of the Medical Underwriters of California. *How MIEC Began in the Medical Liability Crisis of 1975.* Oakland, CA, 1995; Linda O. Prager. "Doctors advised to listen when patients speak on health care." *American Medical News.* Feb. 23, 1998. p. 6.

[33] Paul R. Gross and Noman Levitt. *Higher Superstition: The Academic Left and its Quarrels with Science.* Baltimore and London: Johns Hopkins University Press, 1994, p. 1.

Despite their outward excited aspect, masses are ultra-conservative: in the end masses industriously re-establish the order they enthusiastically destroyed, since for masses, as for any hypnotized subject, the past is infinitely more powerful than the present. Masses tend to be open to suggestion and given to extreme attitudes; yet they are prisoners to traditions, customs and the "ancient unconscious," strongly opposed to over-throwing them. If the goal of a mass is achieved by over-throwing prevailing order, the mass promptly rebuilds all that it demolished.[34] Because the managed care mass movement, called a "revolution" into managed care, goes against the norm such that, if my thesis is correct, once fee-for-service medical practice is destroyed, the mass will go about rebuilding it, or a method very similar to fee-for-service.

"Men, it has been well said, think in herds; it will be seen that they go mad in herds, while they only recover their senses slowly, and one by one.[35]

[34] Serge Moscovici. *The aged of the crowd: A historical treatise on mass psychology.* Translated by J.C. Whitehouse. Cambridge, London, and New York: Cambridge University Press, 1985, p. 114.

[35] Charles Mackay. *Memoirs of Extraordinary Popular Delusions and the Madness of Crowds.* London: Richard Bentley, 1841, reprint. New York: Farrar, Straus and Giroux, 1932, p. xx.

INDEX

Health Care Information Institute, 134

health care resources, 3, 5, 19, 59, 142

health care system, 13, 15, 16, 34, 39, 45, 53, 73, 90, 97, 106, 111, 114, 115, 124, 126

health insurance, 2, 57, 72, 112, 121, 150

health maintenance organizations, 31, 35, 124

Health Net, 64, 72, 96, 104, 105, 123, 132

Health Systems International (HSI), 32, 64, 111

healthy living, 32

higher premiums, 59

high-risk groups, 45

HMO enrollment, 43

HMOs, 3, 4, 6, 12, 15, 16, 20, 22, 27, 28, 32, 36, 39, 41, 44, 45, 50, 60, 64, 65, 68-70, 72, 74-76, 80, 88, 93, 96, 102-104, 106, 108, 110, 112, 113, 115, 126, 135, 136, 146, 150

hold harmless clause, 92

hopelessness, 82, 83

hospital costs, 16, 105

hospitals, 1-3, 5-7, 9, 13, 16-18, 20, 24, 26-28, 30, 31, 44, 48, 52, 60, 63, 68, 70, 72, 79, 82, 92, 95, 102-106, 109, 111, 112, 115, 116, 118, 123, 124, 131, 143, 148

Humana, 59, 60, 61, 104

humanitarian, 38, 90

I

immunizations, 33, 126

imposter term, 18

Imputation of bad design, 40

incentive(s), 3, 5-7, 16, 17, 25, 31, 32, 38, 43, 44, 73, 80, 84, 87, 88, 91, 113, 124, 126, 139, 141, 145

income taxes, 57

incurred-but-not-reported (IBNR), 101, 122

inducement, 71, 86

insolvency, 61, 102, 106, 107, 121-124, 134

insurance industry, 27, 72, 104, 117, 151

insurance, 1-3, 5, 6, 13, 21, 22, 24, 27, 28, 36, 45, 57, 60-62, 65, 67-69, 72-74, 76, 79, 81, 92, 93, 95, 100, 103, 104, 106, 108-110, 112, 115, 117, 121, 122, 125, 133, 134, 139, 141, 143, 148, 150

integrity, 27, 79, 81, 82, 97, 122

intellectual underpinnings, 40, 43, 53, 134, 149

intimidation, 80, 81, 151

investor-owned hospitals, 16

irrelevant conclusion, 18

J

jelly-roll, 60

K

Kaiser *Permanente*, 2, 4, 7, 16, 18, 21-23, 27, 30, 31, 35, 36, 46, 59, 65, 67, 69, 74, 75, 94, 104, 106, 122, 126, 129, 130, 132

knavery, 142

Knox-Keene Act (1975), 11

L

learned helplessness, 129, 130

Legal Center for Patient Protection, 113

legal costs, 5, 92

legislation, 2, 15, 45, 91, 93, 106, 112, 124, 146

liability claims, 92, 93

liability risk, 36

Liberty Plan, 104

life-saving drugs, 4

loss reserve, 122
lower costs, 2, 3, 17, 44, 65, 107
lower premiums, 59, 103

M

M.D. Enterprises of Connecticut
  (MDEC), 64
magazines, 13, 21, 23, 115
magical thinking, 40, 52, 134
major diseases, 3, 99
malpractice, 91, 93, 95, 96, 123, 151
managed care advocates, 2, 7, 54
managed care companies, 4-7, 11, 16,
  18, 19, 24, 27, 31, 33, 46, 48, 52,
  58-63, 65, 68, 69, 71-75, 80-82,
  86, 87, 90, 92-95, 101-107, 109,
  110, 112-114, 116, 118, 121, 123,
  125, 126, 128, 129, 131, 143, 147
managed care enrollment, 43
managed care plans, 1, 4, 11-13, 17,
  22, 24, 28, 32, 34-36, 42, 45, 46,
  48, 49, 51, 52, 57-60, 62, 65, 67,
  69, 70, 72, 74, 79-82, 86, 89-96,
  102-106, 108, 110, 113, 115, 116,
  121-128, 134, 141, 148, 149
managed competition, 71, 72, 110,
  118, 139, 141
market solution, 118, 126
market-driven, 65, 73
marketing consultants, 44
market-oriented health care, 53
Maxicare Health Plan, 101
Medicaid, 2, 3, 82, 104, 109, 110,
  113, 125, 148, 149
medical care, x, 1, 2, 5-7, 18-21, 27,
  30, 31, 37, 43-46, 48-50, 52, 53,
  61, 65, 67, 68, 72, 80, 95-97, 99,
  102, 104, 106, 109, 111, 114, 116,
  118, 119, 125, 127, 130, 134, 141-
  143, 145, 147, 149, 151
Medical Code of Ethics, 68
medical costs, 3, 12, 25, 31, 44, 61,
  99, 126, 142, 147
medical ethics, 71

medical insurance plans, 1, 143
medical judgment, 90, 91, 95
medical liability, 27, 92
medical necessity, 72
medical personnel, 133, 149
medical record, 37
medical research, 39, 44, 105
medical resources, 45, 50, 143
medical services, 1-3, 5, 11, 13, 19,
  44, 45, 59, 60, 67, 70, 72, 81, 99,
  109, 115, 116, 128, 129, 136, 143,
  144, 151
medical treatments, 4, 39
Medicare, 2- 4, 12, 13, 16, 32, 35, 46,
  59, 67, 70-72, 76, 82, 99, 104,
  105, 108-110, 113, 122, 124, 125,
  129, 134, 144, 148, 149
men and women-of-words, 42
mergers, 11, 13, 16, 17, 61, 62, 102,
  111
miracle of capitation, 134
miracle(s), 53, 54, 134, 136, 142
missive regression, 76
multiple sclerosis, 50
mysterious absurdity, 21, 30
myth, 53, 54, 57, 85, 106

N

national health, 45, 72
New England Journal of Medicine, 4,
  7, 13, 17, 20, 22, 23, 27, 35, 40,
  41, 43- 45, 51, 60, 62, 67, 69-72,
  76, 79-82, 88, 89, 97, 99, 103-105,
  109, 111, 113, 114, 125, 126, 130,
  139, 141, 143, 146, 147
newspapers, 21, 99, 115
nurse practitioners, 37
nursing home costs, 144

O

obstetrician(s), 37, 96
Official Malefactor's Screen, 75
open access plans, 104

W

Washington, 3, 12, 32, 39, 44, 60, 61,
     70, 88, 135, 136, 146
Wellness Programs, 31
withhold, 68, 80, 86, 101, 112

working the float, 70
World War II, 3, 39, 144

Z

zealots, ix, 73, 135, 142